Reclaim Your Youth:
Growing Younger After 40

by

Richard Sullivan

Copyright 2009 Richard Sullivan

Montgomery Ewing Publishers

www.discoveringhawaii.com

dedicated to my friend-since-we-was-babies,

Steve Whelan

who, even though we live on opposite sides of the world,

is always there for me.

Chapter 1 / *page 4*
Only You Can Decide How Old You Are

Chapter 2 / *page 12*
Growing Younger After 40

Chapter 3 / *page 32*
Strength Training: New Muscle, New Bone

Chapter 4 / *page 62*
The Open Secrets Of Strength Training

Chapter 5 / *page 98*
Your Strength Training Workout Routine: Exercise Menu and Advice

Chapter 6 / *page 122*
My Workout

Chapter 7 / *page 128*
The Simple Reclaim Your Youth Diet

Chapter 8 / *page 134*
What Do I Eat?

Chapter 9 / *page 150*
22 Things You Can Do Right Now To Take Back Your Youth

Chapter 1
Only You Can Decide How Old You Are

If you're standing in the bookstore right now reading this, and wondering whether you should buy this book, maybe I can save you some money:

—There is no magic pill, and there never will be.

—There is no revolutionary diet.

—There are no effortless exercises.

Reclaiming, or taking back your youth requires as much diligence, persistence and continuous effort as anything else that has been worth pursuing in your life, such as your career, or a primary relationship.

Although in the last chapter this book outlines quite a few ways to immediately make yourself younger, Reclaim Your Youth is not about a fast and easy quick-fix. It's about taking back control in those precious few areas of your life where it is actually possible to do so.

We have little control over our lives... our friends, lovers, family. People can move away, find someone else, or die.

How much control do we have over our job, career, or business? We might get laid off, people can stop buying our products or services, or, as we have already experienced, the economy can suddenly tank. Whatever we own can be taken away from us.

In virtually every aspect of our lives, attaining satisfaction depends heavily on the cooperation or permission of others, with one exception: our own body.

Our body is the only thing in life we truly control. Only we decide what we eat and how much, what we drink or inhale; whether we exercise and in what ways, and how much. We control all these things. No one else has a say.

The body we inhabit right now, the way it looks, and the state of health it's in, is the precise result of all our past decisions. Any change we make in our decisions today will be newly reflected in the way our bodies look, feel, and move tomorrow.

What this means is, once we make up our minds to do so, we really can turn back the hands of time, *right now*, literally. There are dozens of things we can do to turn things around, some of them easy and immediate, others more challenging and longer-term. But nothing comes close to possessing the all-encompassing power to change our lives so completely as does strength training.

Taking control over our own aging process is the ultimate in self-empowerment. Personal trainers, plastic surgeons and anti-aging gurus may all have their place, but ultimately we alone are responsible for slowing, halting, and reversing aspects of our own aging process.

Believing that we can't do it without "expert" assistance deprives us of one of the most powerful anti-aging strategies we have at our disposal: our independence.

Take Back Your Youth 101

In my role as coach you might find me a tad unsympathetic at times. Blame it on the fact that I was a personal trainer in LA who, for too much of that time, felt more like a baby sitter. LA is the place where everybody feels compelled to look great, but too few feel compelled to actually do the work required to look great.

On the bright side, I am empathetic, encouraging, and highly optimistic, because I've been there myself. I've struggled with inertia and lack of direction. I've been lazy more than I've been enthused. I've had major problems getting my butt out of the chair during certain periods of my life. I worked out for way too long without any coherent exercise plan, eating plan, or specific goal, and therefore didn't accomplish what I'd hoped. Along the way I learned and sought advice from media materials and from individuals who had already accomplished what I wanted to. I read and studied and listened, and little by little applied what I learned, and was happily surprised to see that when I set a goal, decided to go after in a focused manner, and stuck with it, making it part of my lifestyle, I began to excel physically in a way few people my age have.

Above all, I'm a good coach because I'm successful at doing this, both for myself and for others, and have been steadily increasing my knowledge and experience for forty years. And I get better at getting better with every passing day.

What Does "Happiness" Mean To You?

When people describe what happiness means to them…what it would take to make them happy right now at this moment…their responses are highly individual. For some it might mean meeting the love of their life. For others it would be having enough money to pay all their bills and travel the world experiencing new things, or remodeling the house, or being able to spend more quality time with their kids or grandchildren. But all of these responses have one given in common: that we will be healthy and able enough for these things to even be possible.

If you have breathing difficulties, tire easily while climbing stairs, or can't run 50 yards to save yourself, your quality of life is already diminished. If you are sick or disabled with diabetes, heart disease, cancer, or stroke, your chances and opportunities for finding the perfect lover, spending quality time with the grandkids, taking on a months-long remodeling project, or traveling the world experiencing everything new and exciting are not that promising.

Every desire for our happiness depends on two things: good health, and physical strength. A strong and healthy body is necessary for performing well sexually so we can win over and keep our dream mate. A strong and healthy body is necessary for running after, playing with, and most importantly, protecting your kids or grandkids while they are in your charge. A strong and healthy body is necessary for the rigors of traveling the world or tackling new and exciting things, like that remodeling project.

Strength is something that people choose to lose as they age, because there is no scientific justification for this loss.

Humans never lose their capacity to build new muscle and bone, nor to significantly strengthen what they already have… not even seniors who are well into their 90s. If we are not intentionally building new muscle after age 30, then we're losing it by default, day by day.

It is curious that we focus so intensely on our face or hair and how others may be judging our wrinkles or bald spot, while ignoring the fact that the true measure of youth is our strength, agility, health, and the physical ability to enjoy everything life has to offer.

Men obsess over hair loss and spend a fortune trying to combat that, yet they do not obsess one bit over muscle loss. Men feel less virile and less masculine when they lose their hair, but how strange not to feel less virile and less masculine when their muscles evaporate. Along with muscle loss, men lose their manly strength, manly sex drive and sexual ability, their sexual and overall attractiveness to others, and manly physique and presence.

Women too obsess over hair and nails and all forms of superficiality while ignoring the one thing that will truly mark them as youthful and attractive, and that is a strong, tight, agile physique. A healthy person looks good and projects high self esteem, an unhealthy person does not. Trying to become more attractive via unhealthy or superficial cosmetic methods means literally taking one step forward and two steps back.

Good looks go hand in hand with, and are the result of, good health and physical strength. Once you make peace with your body rather than waging war against it, you will succeed. Once you supplement your desire to look younger, or to have the perfect body, with the sincere desire to do what's right for your health and well being, everything else will fall into place.

Once you stop seeing your body as the enemy and the obstacle to happiness, and begin to view it as the vehicle capable of transporting you to realms you've only yet dreamed of, its shape, size and abilities will begin to change almost effortlessly.

In an interview a couple of years ago, Oprah Winfrey said that it wasn't until she weighed 237 lbs. and was listening to the announcer while attending a Mike Tyson fight that she realized she weighed more than the heavyweight champion of the world. That was her epiphany.

After years of struggling with her weight, she abruptly decided to make friends with her physical heart instead, and promised her heart that she would do everything she could to help it do its job pumping blood, transporting oxygen and giving her life.

It wasn't until she embraced the idea of optimum health and the promises that mobility, vigor and longevity hold, rather than obsessing about having a perfect body, that her entire attitude toward nutrition and exercise changed. And lo and behold, she ended up getting the kind of body she always wanted in the bargain anyway. Her years of weight battles and diets got her nowhere, but that one second it took her to surrender to the service of her own health and well-being completely changed her body from the inside out.

Then, in 2008, she again ballooned up to 200 lbs., admitting her diet and exercise regimen had somehow gone out the window. By 2008, Oprah's friendship with her heart was apparently on the rocks.

Stay tuned.

What's Wrong With Me Anyway?

We could spend a couple of chapters of this book delving into our childhood traumas and all the nasty people who screwed us up so bad that we ended up using food, alcohol, drugs and nicotine to mask our hurt, calm our fears and create barriers between us and the rest of the scary world, but then we'd still end up in the same place anyway: the place where we need to make a change. So let's skip ahead and get right down to the part where we decide to stop the self destructive behaviors that stonewall our happiness and rob us of our youth.

Some wizened soul has said, "Getting older is not for sissies". All of us are guilty of complaining, which if you've noticed, hasn't gotten us anywhere. So let's get busy with actually turning our lives around in the right direction.

Chapter 2
Growing Younger After 40

In recent years a wonderful and exciting change has swept over the science of aging. Destructive beliefs about getting older, rooted in hopelessness and negative tradition and embraced as truth for millennia, have been challenged —and dismissed. Inspiring new scientific discoveries continue to be made almost daily concerning the ways our bodies can and do repair themselves, despite decades of damage. These discoveries are responsible for the optimistic turnaround in the way our aging population has now begun to view itself and its future.

Perhaps it's just embedded in our genetics for us to bulldoze ahead through life as if we are indestructible, despite the troubling image of that stranger we may see in the full-length mirror right after our shower. Ignoring that disquieting reflection, we continue to insist on believing that whenever we get around to mending our ways we can actually undo most of the damage we've inflicted upon our bodies.

So, can we really? Or are we just kidding ourselves?

It used to be unimaginable that someone past the age of 40 could create a body virtually indistinguishable from that of someone in their 20s. But paging through any bodybuilding magazine at the supermarket today will reveal it's not just *possible*, but relatively common.

Only recently has it begun to sink into people's consciousness that building a healthy, strong and attractive body has little to do with chronological age, and is achievable well past the age of 40. It is no longer possible to blindly ignore the thousands of people who have done this very thing just so that we can justify our own life choices, or to believe that only Hollywood stars are privy to the "secrets" or have the resources to hold back the march of time.

There is indeed a lot more fact than fiction to our not-so-egotistical belief that we can undo a significant amount of the damage that we have visited upon ourselves through our neglect and bad habits…indeed, even that caused by decades of chain smoking, for example. It has been proven beyond any doubt that the positive effects of cessation of smoking most significantly the ceasing of damaging chronic inflammation begin within *minutes* after stopping, and not years down the line, as most people seem to still believe.

Chronological vs. Biological Aging

There are two types of aging that we experience: chronological aging and biological aging.

Chronological aging is something we all do at the same rate. After 60 years have passed, we're all 60 years older. But biological aging is far less rigid and predictable. Biologically, after 60 years have passed, one person can look and feel 40, while another can look and feel 75. Most of us don't "get old" just because time passes. We actually work very hard at wearing our bodies out and diminishing our health. In our quest to escape our problems and cope with our day-to-day stress, we continually make decisions that negatively affect how quickly and how significantly we age.

Our negative choices involving food, physical activity and intoxicants contribute overwhelmingly to our individual aging rate.

Until recently, only the ever-elusive Fountain Of Youth was thought to be the answer to restoring our bodies to vigorous form and function. For centuries man has fantasized about finding this fictional solution to his inevitable fate. The stubborn truth is that our ongoing unwise eating, drinking, inhaling, and physical inactivity decisions have been responsible for robbing us of much of our health, looks and strength. We have to make changes in these problem areas if we expect to turn back the clock and take back our youth.

The Fountain Of Youth idea, and its closely related *Magic Pill* and *Secret Hollywood Formula* cousins, illustrates our deep-seated desire to believe in a quick and easy fix. Taking back our youth will never be as simple as doing one thing, like drinking from a fountain, taking a pill, or discovering a secret.

There is no single answer to reclaiming renewed health, strength or beauty. Since there are many factors that contribute to attractiveness, health and strength, there are dozens of different options we have to choose from to work on so we can achieve our ultimate goal. The more constructive behaviors that we can adopt to replace the destructive ones, the younger and healthier we will appear, feel, and actually become. Taken together, the way we eat, think, move, react, stand, communicate, and sleep will give us back a body we can be truly proud of, the health we fear we are losing, and the strength we need to accomplish every new goal that lies ahead. Reclaiming our youth is a holistic, ongoing endeavor involving a lot of little baby steps and a few well-timed challenging leaps.

Muscle And Bone Are The Very Foundations Of Our Being

The muscle that is our heart continually pumps blood through our bodies, while other muscles hold our skeleton together and make our every move possible. Muscle is the engine that drives our immune system and our ability to fight every kind of disease, from the common cold to cancer. Muscle burns fat.

Muscle is the house where our metabolism lives. The pernicious loss of our precious lean muscle mass over the years means that we now get fat on the same amount of food that used to keep us slim just a few years ago. Muscle loss also means we get sick more easily, more often and for a longer period of time, and take longer to recover.

Our skeleton is the foundation of our entire being. Upon accidentally walking into the furniture, strong bone makes all the difference between a sore shin and a life-altering compound fracture. Together, muscle and bone make everything we do in our daily lives possible. Most of us know what it's like to be sidelined by a leg, foot, or toe injury, and how intrusive that is on our ability to accomplish all that we need to during our day.

Imagine how your abilities would be altered if suddenly every muscle in your body were weakened and diminished, along with your bone density as well. The term "shrunken", which is a term associated with the slow, almost imperceptible loss we are all now experiencing, is too inadequate to describe such a devastating loss. After shrinking, a sweater will still weigh the same as it did before, even though the size changes. But when muscle and bone shrink, they are gone. Their size, their weight and their density have evaporated. Yet, we still have the ability to reclaim them.

Starting around age 30, the very core of our physical being literally begins to dematerialize.

Beginning at age 30, we lose an astonishing 7% of our total lean muscle mass each passing decade thereafter. As a result of that muscle loss, we also lose a significant amount of strength, our capacity to efficiently burn calories, our youthful body shape, form, contour and movement, and our ability to resist and conquer illnesses.

Some men and women may come to suffer from the chronic disease called osteoporosis. But as we age, everyone experiences a thinning and weakening of the bones unless they are actively working to combat it.

We now have scientific proof that we can actually reclaim decades' worth of lost muscle and bone, the very underpinnings of a strong, youthful body. Even though we fitness professionals have witnessed this very regeneration phenomenon for decades among our own clients, most of the general public has clung to the false and hopeless belief that, whatever their age, it was "too late" for them to turn back the clock by rebuilding lost muscle and bone, and along with it, youthful looks and movement.

Tufts University's Ground-breaking Findings

Revolutionary research carried out at Tufts University in the 1990s scientifically proved once and for all that rebuilding lost muscle and bone is within everyone's capability. Indeed, it is possible for people to be stronger and physically more attractive even in their senior years than they were in their youth.

The ground-breaking research by Miriam E. Nelson PhD and colleagues at Tufts has proven what many of us in the fitness community already had knowledge of anecdotally, but up until recently had no hard scientific evidence to support: that many of the weaknesses and maladies blamed on aging are in actuality caused by the insidious loss of muscle and bone, which in turn are caused almost exclusively by lifestyle choices.

Dr. Nelson's studies confirmed that we never lose our ability to replenish dissipated muscle and bone, or to build anew. The fact that a man or woman in their 80s can be in better physical shape than ever been before is an astonishing concept, yet entirely possible. After all, people in their 80s who are running marathons now, but who were couch potatoes in their 30s, are not genetic anomalies. True, they are currently the exception to the rule, but they certainly don't have to be. Anyone in reasonably good health can exponentially improve his or her overall health, strength, physical beauty, and quality of life, to paraphrase the Nike slogan, by Just Doing It.

Scientists, a very curious species who doubt or ignore their own anecdotal experiences and observations until some colleague publishes a paper to support them, formerly believed that loss of strength, muscle and bone were just part and parcel of getting older.

In a report published in 1990 in the Journal of the American Medical association [JAMA], a Tufts research group led by Maria Fiatarone MD conducted a study with elderly residents of a senior citizens home employing weight training to see if strength and muscle size could be achieved by the extremely aged.

In this case, four men and six women between the ages of 86 and 96 dependably showed up three times a week for eight weeks in the nursing home's exercise room. The weight training machines used were the same as those found in commercial gyms and health clubs.

The results were unexpected and quite extraordinary. As might be surmised, these subjects were frail human beings. All suffered from at least two serious chronic diseases, including heart disease, osteoporosis and diabetes. Most got around with the help of walkers and canes and a number of the subjects could not even get out of a chair without assistance.

In only eight weeks these very elderly people increased their strength by an astonishing average of 175%. In a test for balance and walking speed they increased their scores 48%, and two of the subjects were able to walk again without the aid of their canes.

We humans are not predestined to become hopelessly fragile as we age. Among the elderly, loss of strength, loss of balance, and repeated falls are all related directly to loss of muscle and bone mass, which are completely preventable and to an astonishing degree, reversible.

Science has proven that strength, agility, muscle shape, physical attractiveness and even our sense of balance are all recoverable commodities, no matter what our age or strength level at the present time.

Why We Need To Reclaim Our Youth

If you're past 40 you already have noticed a number of the differences, many of them troubling, between the 20 year-old you and the over-40-year-old you. Everything from a body that bears little resemblance to what it once was, to bleeding gums and aching knees remind us each day that aging not only isn't much fun, but has a lot of undesirable side effects we'd rather do without.

As we said earlier, everyone ages at the same speed chronologically, but biologically we age at different rates. Aging is actually a choice, biologically speaking. Our biological age is governed by two factors: our genetics, which we have more control over than people like to think, and our lifestyle choices, which we have complete control over.

The best genetics on the planet cannot overcome damaging lifestyle choices. However, great lifestyle choices can overwhelmingly prevail over inopportune genetics.

Type-2 diabetes is overwhelmingly a lifestyle disease. 90% of all type-2 diabetes sufferers never *need* develop the disease at all. Their lifestyle choices and damaging habits bring on pre-diabetes condition, and continuing or escalating these same habits over as long as a decade allow their pre-diabetes to develop into full-blown diabetes. That's a heck of a lot of lead-time to reconsider changing one's debilitating ways! Type-2 diabetes doesn't develop overnight. It takes many. many years of unwise nutrition and inactivity choices to develop.

Scientists estimate that we ourselves create 70% of all the maladies associated with aging through our determination to continue, and even accelerate, damaging lifestyle choices.

Puzzlingly, most people prefer to believe that aging is something that just happens to us and over which we have no control. They will fight the idea that any dietary changes, physical fitness activity or the surrendering of destructive habits will make a difference. They will look older sooner, become chronically ill with a greater number of diseases earlier in life, and die younger on average than those who understand and implement the simple rationale behind goal-oriented nutrition and fitness.

On the other hand, those individuals who acknowledge responsibility for their past choices, are willing to substitute new behaviors for old, and accept the scientifically confirmed idea that it's never too late to make significant changes will be the most successful at reclaiming their youth.

Some people race toward old age as if it were a sprint, while others pace themselves, marathon fashion. It seems by the sprinters' choices, they just can't wait to get there fast enough. They boast about their artery-clogging fat intake, joke about their lack of physical fitness, and light up yet another cigarette.

They are condescendingly amused by others who work diligently to improve their health, strength and attractiveness, disparagingly referring to these odd creatures who are crazy enough to care for themselves as health *nuts*. They explain that they are unwilling to "deprive" themselves because they've "earned it", and because "life is too short"...and indeed, for most of them, it will be.

Enjoying life to its fullest means different things to different people. For some it means eating whatever they want whenever they want it, never physically exerting themselves any more than necessary, or freely indulging in alcohol, tobacco and prescription or illegal drugs at will.

To others it means having a body they can be proud of and to be secure in the knowledge that it can perform as needed, when needed, painlessly. It means being able to run from danger or to quickly climb out of a car window if need be. It means knowing they have the ability to save themselves and their loved ones in an emergency that requires physical strength, agility and speed. It means getting older without being weighed down by chronic illness or disability and the deep depression and hopelessness that often accompanies these conditions.

Most Of Us Have No Idea Just How Bad We Feel

The human body has an almost surreal ability to adjust and accommodate even near-fatal physical maladies. During the worst years of the AIDS epidemic of the 1980s and early 1990s, physicians marveled at how many times a single patient could recover from a series of fungal, bacterial and viral infections, any one of which could have killed a perfectly healthy individual. How could people so emaciated, weakened and damaged recover from not just one, but a series of potentially fatal episodes? As far as I know, no one has ever formally studied this particular phenomenon, in which it seems lies valuable answers for the treatment of all human disease.

Due to this remarkable ability our bodies possess to adjust to the most adverse of conditions, few people are conscious of how physically unwell they presently feel.

The hard truth is that we middle- and senior-aged people, in addition to having already lost a significant amount of muscle mass and bone density, have a long history of wear-and-tear and bad habits that have exacted an ongoing toll on our mobility, strength, health, agility, and energy. Most of us are literally walking around in a dull, less-than-well state without being fully aware of just how poorly we feel. *We've just gotten used to it* gradually as we allowed it to creep subtly and diabolically into our lives. We accept it as normal… as if it were an inevitable outcome of getting older.

The ongoing, almost imperceptible loss of muscle strength and size does not become critical in most people until their senior years. By that time it can reach a point where an individual begins to experience an unsettling sense of panic related to the physical unsteadiness they experience due to the loss of strength and balance. Disturbing new thoughts and experiences can lead to unwelcome personal dilemmas, such as damaged self confidence, overall fear and anxiety about the future, and social withdrawal.

For many people, denial of aging might manifest itself in the acceleration of their existing bad habits, or adopting new ones to mask and soothe apprehension concerning their perceived loss of youth and ability. Overindulgence in favorite foods, alcohol, nicotine and prescription or recreational drugs are the most common methods of masking pain, both physical and emotional. Eventually, though, the problems will snowball to a point where they must be faced head on, or the results for the individual can become irreversible and catastrophic.

Today we know far more about the repair, reclamation and rejuvenation of the human body than ever before, and instead of dulling our senses with comfort substances to keep from having to face the loss of our youth, we now have the tools to set about recapturing it.

For many people, more than just reclaiming the youthful attributes and abilities they once had, they can actually become physically better today in many ways than they ever were in their chronological youth.

The Reasons Why We Need To Remain Biologically Young

It's no secret that aging brings with it the specter of some truly frightening possibilities most of us claim we would do just about anything to avoid. However, the damage that the bulk of the adult population is willfully visiting upon themselves right this minute contradicts that claim. Denial can be the only logical explanation for this curious self-destruction. Over 60% of all adults in the US are overweight, but the senior population is the fattest, most unfit population of all, and certainly by far the most vulnerable to the destructive effects of obesity.

It is not irrational to fear aging, especially for those who are beginning to question their negative lifestyle choices. The desire to alleviate our fears can be a powerful impetus in propelling us toward taking action against biological aging by making new choices It is difficult to enjoy one's longevity if chronically ill, disabled or bedridden. Quality of life is far more precious than the length of one's lifespan. Living longer means little if we're in too much pain —physical, emotional and spiritual— to enjoy those extra years.

For those people who ignore their physical health, advancing years and medical crises like heart disease, stroke, cancer, and diabetes will be exacerbated by inevitable feelings of hopelessness, regret, and depression.

Those individuals struggling financially in addition to facing one or more serious health events can multiply the weight of their tribulations tenfold.

The bottom line is this: rational people do not ever want to go there, and will begin taking steps to avoid it, now.

Saving Ourselves And The Ones We Love

After hearing firsthand accounts and seeing vivid images of horrific events, all of us have imagined what it might be like to be in some terrible situation, like a fire, automobile or airline crash, or terrorist attack. Could we make it out? Perhaps more importantly, could we also get our loved ones out safely?

The weight loss and fitness industries are multi-billion dollar enterprises, and the number one driving force behind them is personal vanity.

And that's okay.

There's absolutely nothing wrong with wanting to look great. The additional rewards that come from being attractive will shower down upon you each and every day.

A distant second in most people's minds when it comes to fitness and weight loss is wellness. They know they will stand a better chance of maintaining good health, and living longer in good health, rather than in infirmity, if they lose excess weight and become physically fit.

But perhaps the most important, yet least considered aspect of being physically strong and fit, is the ability to remove ourselves and loved ones from danger…to save ourselves in a life-threatening situation.

Can you fit through the car window if the door can't be opened and the vehicle is submerging or on fire? Could you bring your children out with you? Can you swiftly make it down, or up, multiple flights of stairs to escape mortal danger? Can you scramble up a riverbank, scale a wall, run 3 or 4 blocks at top speed without tripping? Do you dismiss these scenarios, believing it will never happen to you?

When the spectre of calamities such as these enter our minds, most of us try to banish them as quickly as possible, but it is important to imagine yourself in your own home, vehicle or workplace in just such a situation, and then formulate an escape route or plan. And then imagine that if that route were blocked, what would your alternate plan be?

Being physically strong means that you have the ability, and the *agility*, to transport yourself down the stairway, out the window, or over the fence and away from danger.

September 11

Vividly recounted survivor stories from the September 11 terrorist attacks disturbingly illustrated how mere seconds made the difference between life and death for scores of people. Dozens of individuals later recounted how they were just one or two seconds inside the window of opportunity for escape as debris crashed down, floors collapsed, or fires raged.

How many deceased or now-disabled individuals do you think might have been just one or two seconds *outside* their window of opportunity? How many were just *one or two precious seconds short* of being able to save themselves? Who knows how many died because of their physical inability to flee quickly enough, to surmount obstacles, to climb or run, because their escape was compromised by their weight or poor level of fitness? The few seconds that could have made the difference between life and death for these people may have been lost due to these factors.

Only strength training builds significant strength, muscle and bone. Aerobics, yoga, jogging, swimming, power-walking and the like are all terrific fitness exercise, but they don't build significant muscle, strength, or bone. The dictionary definition of significant is *meaningful*, and meaningful means *"that which will make an important difference."*

It's clear that the wrong generation is in the gyms and health clubs. The twenty and thirty year olds still retain most of their genetically-bestowed muscle mass, yet there they are, pumping away, creating more.

But it is us geezers —oops— I mean us middle-agers and seniors who have lost major amounts of both muscle and bone as we've aged who should be beating a path to our local gym, or strength training at home.

Getting older regrettably *does* mean getting shorter, smaller and weaker for the majority of people, but it doesn't have to be that way.

Your rate and degree of aging is a choice, and choosing to instead become stronger and more vital as we get older is a very powerful option that is within everyone's capability. It is the fountain of youth that man has searched for since the beginning of time.

Fear

Physical weaknesses can dictate how we live and alter our lives in literally hundreds of conscious, unconscious, pervasive, and invasive ways. Our lack of strength slowly shrinks our world and pens us in. Our choices are diminished and our joy substantially lessened.

We ultimately begin making decisions *to not do* certain things or *to not go* certain places based of our lack of strength, our fears, and consequently, our ability. People can go so far as to become housebound due to both rational and irrational trepidations, such as fear of physical attack, fear of falling, fear of being chased by dogs or other apprehensions that have accumulated and festered due to a prolonged period of diminishing strength and the self-doubts that accompany that.

Many people haven't even made the connection yet between their puzzling new fears and hesitations, and the fact that their recent lifestyle limitations are directly related to their reduced physical ability and resulting diminished self-confidence.

All too often people will say "It must be because I'm getting old" to explain away something that's limiting them that in reality has far more to do with diminished physical strength and ability that it does aging. Increased physical strength is equally as powerful a benefit of adopting a strength training regimen as is newfound attractiveness and enhanced health.

The strength which allows us to face the world head-on or to flee danger is just one kind of physical strength. Another kind is the strength our bodies develop to battle, reverse and conquer illness.

Diabetes is but one example where it has been proven that

increased fitness has a profound effect on reversing symptoms. 17 million Americans are currently suffering from diabetes. In addition, another 16 million are on the verge, suffering from what is called pre-diabetes condition, caused in large part by the increase in obesity in the US. These people will most likely develop full-blown diabetes within ten years, but few actually need to.

Recent studies have shown that the symptoms of pre-diabetes can be reversed. A government clinical trial called the Diabetes Prevention Program has shown that those designated as pre-diabetics can help prevent the onset of Type-2 diabetes by engaging in a moderate, 30 minute per day, 5 days a week exercise program, and by cutting down on fat and calories in their diet.

The study was conducted with 3,000 overweight people and it was found that by losing only 5% to 7% of their total bodyweight —which for a 250 lb. person only amounts to 12.5 lbs. to 17.5 lbs.— that they cut their diabetes risk *in half*. This is a much better result than any currently available medication can achieve.

For a 250 lb. person, dropping to approximately 235 lbs. is a small price to pay for such a huge impact on one's health. Diabetes is the number one cause of blindness in adults, and a major cause of heart attack, stroke, and loss of limbs by amputation. Adopting a *challenging* —as opposed to *moderate*— ongoing fitness regimen, and reducing weight to near-normal levels will allow most people to cross diabetes completely off their list forever.

Diabetes is such a hideous disease, and so easily preventable for most people, that it is beyond reason that any human on the verge of contracting it would reject the chance to reverse their horrendous fate. Yet, millions continue to do exactly that. Overweight people over the age of 40 should be screened for pre-diabetes during their annual medical exam, but for black people in particular this is especially critical.

Physicians' Dilemma

Adding to the long list of problems and drawbacks associated with aging unhealthfully, there is a severe and escalating shortage of physicians specializing in geriatrics in the United States. Considering the vast numbers of rapidly aging baby boomers, this shortage is very disquieting.

The elderly are not an attractive patient population to most physicians for many reasons. Medicare payments to doctors have been repeatedly reduced over the years, forcing doctors to make the difficult choice of either dropping Medicare patients altogether, or taking a financial loss.

Doctors need to spend more time with geriatric patients than with others, but are not only *not paid more* for this time, but in the example of Medicare cutbacks, are actually paid less.

Medical residents who might otherwise be drawn to geriatrics have the very real quandary of trying to figure out how they could possibly repay gargantuan med school loans when geriatric care pays so poorly compared to specialties like cardiology or gastroenterology.

Because many younger doctors through the eyes of youth see senior patients' medical problems as intractable, they often may not be as aggressive in determining the genesis of a problem or in their treatment of the problem itself. Doctors who are focused on a successful outcome and who are driven by a desire to make patients feel better, if not cure them completely, can be uncomfortable treating patients for whom they see no cure or significant improvement ahead.

In other words, some older people die before their time simply because their illnesses are not detected as early or treated as aggressively as the same illness would be in a younger person. A doctor may tell an 80 year old that his knee pain is due to his age, "so deal with it", whereas the same doctor would search for a way to treat a 20-year-old presenting with the exact same symptoms.

What Is The Definition Of "Youth", Anyway?

For some, youth is displayed by an absence of wrinkles, an attitude, a certain body image, or even a way of walking.

But youth is more than just outward appearance. Youth is more than a fit-looking body. Youth is a way of moving, talking, thinking, anticipating the future, working toward new goals, caring for and about one's self and loved ones. Youth is good health and an absence of self-destructive behaviors.

Youth is self-focused, but not self-centered.

Youth is a feeling and a mood and a way of looking at the world and its possibilities in an optimistic way. Youth means not believing that the best of you exists only in past memories. Youth is being more enthused about tomorrow than about yesterday.

This book's message is Reclaim Your Youth. It's about cultivating nostalgia for your *future*, rather than your past.

Chapter 3
Strength Training: New Muscle, New Bone.

> *"If I knew I was going to live this long, I would have taken a whole lot better care of myself."*
> —Mickey Mantel

The terms strength training, resistance training and weight training are all interchangeable. We make use of all three terms in this book, but they all mean the same thing.

Most men have very little problem with the concept of building muscle, but since many women think of strength and muscle as unfeminine, they seem to respond better to the term resistance training. The truth is, ladies, without strength you can't pick up toddlers —or have as much fun creating them— rearrange the living room furniture, or remove yourself or your loved ones from danger.

Whatever your gender, strength training can take your body to undreamed of frontiers of attractiveness, ability, agility and mobility.

Despite protests from those suffering the consequences of self-neglect and the silly complaints that society and the media place too much emphasis on youth and attractive people, our own experience and common sense tell us differently.

All of us have experienced the favorable reactions of others when we have looked especially good because of weight loss, a change in hairstyle, or new clothing. These favorable reactions, which bolster our ego and brighten our lives, need never cease. They can continue coming our way for the rest of our days.

Miracles Will Happen.

We all know what muscle does for a man's appearance, but what about women?

What actually makes a woman's legs or arms or back *beautiful* is muscle. Well-toned, well-maintained muscle. Increased attractiveness is just one of the incredible benefits that weight training brings. Weight training will make you more attractive.

Weight training will not just make you feel younger; it will actually make you younger. Strength training reverses the aging process.

Weight training not only stops bone loss, but creates brand-new bone, increases tendon and ligament strength and size, and enhances the beauty and size of your muscle exactly in those places where you need or want it most.

Weight training will ease depression or dissipate it altogether.

Weight training builds self esteem, imbues general feelings of well being, eases our fears about growing older, diminishes or stops insomnia, and allows us to eat favorite foods more often.

Weight training reinforces our immune system, allowing us to more vigorously fight off everything from colds to cancer. Strength training increases physical energy to the point where you might want to go out dancing for the first time in years, instead of sitting home watching *Dancing With The Stars*.

Best of all, weight training helps renew our sex life by stimulating our libido and increasing our vigor and stamina. Weight training makes us more attractive to potential sex partners. Weight training strengthens the muscles that allow us to attain and maintain specific pleasurable sexual positions. And that increased energy and staying power will allow the sex act to last longer and be performed more vigorously and in a more controlled manner.

Weight training increases our energy stores. Although it might seem a contradiction, since we already know from personal experience that lifting and moving heavy objects can zap our energy and cause our muscles to ache the next day, this is actually true. You will find at the beginning of your program that *you will* feel somewhat drained and stiff, because your muscles, unaccustomed to this new routine, will be tired and your newly-awakened body will ache a little. But after your first 4 to 6 workouts, wonderful changes will begin to occur.

Your body, owing to 2 million years of evolution, will become accustomed to the stress of strength training by *adapting*. Adapting to the stress. Adapting to the weight load by growing new muscle and increasing in strength. And that stiffness you feel, and will continue to feel on those days when you push yourself a little harder, is what growing muscle feels like as it is repairing itself from the stresses of weight training and builds new strength to better handle the increased load you have placed on it.

Perhaps the best weight training perk of all is that muscle actually burns fat. Even while you're asleep, 24/7. The more muscle you build and strengthen, the faster your metabolism, and the greater your fat-burning capabilities.

Although these claims may sound like some late-night infomercial come-on, they are all scientifically true.

The Unbreakable Triangle

Whether your main goal in following the principles laid out in this book is to either become more attractive, or healthier, or physically stronger, *all three* of those benefits will be yours *automatically*.

Think of strength training as an unbreakable triangle, with one side representing attractiveness, the second representing health, and the third representing strength.

Strength, health and attractiveness are equal and inseparable components of the same strength training triangle, no matter which of the three might be your primary goal.

Magic Pill

It not only seems that the majority of people are waiting around for science to come up with a pill that will give them many of the benefits that weight training does, but polls have shown that many people actually believe such a pill is right around the corner.

Putting off getting into shape because you think such a pill will come on the market sometime soon is akin to planning on quitting your job even though your home is about to be foreclosed on because you're convinced you're going to win the lottery soon.

Many people are enduring pain and suffering, weakness and feelings of helplessness that would quickly cease if they would simply adopt an ongoing basic weight training program. Even if science were able to make a magic pill that would allow us to eat whatever we want and still have a slim body, we still would have none of the glowing toned muscle or the bone strength benefits that come from strength training.

Fear Of Muscle

Women especially seem to have a hard time grappling with the idea of getting stronger, as many equate muscle with masculinity. Every woman has 333 muscles in her body, the same as a man. The heart that pumps your blood and keeps you alive is a muscle. Muscle keeps your lungs drawing breath. Muscle is what holds your breasts up, and as this foundation weakens and atrophies, your breasts go with it.

Women fill their blouses and jackets with shoulder pads to mimic muscle, but resist actually building larger shoulders so they can have the same impressive look naturally. Women wear high heels to make their calf muscles look bigger and shapelier, but won't weight train to actually make their calves bigger and shapelier, a look they could show off round-the-clock. High heels elongate the legs by flexing the thighs, yet women don't seem to want to put forth the effort to strength train so that their thighs can always look beautiful, even when shoeless. Some women wear foundation garments to hold in bulges that are due in large part to unchallenged, soft, weak midsection muscles, instead of working out to harden, strengthen and tone these muscles so they didn't have to pry themselves in and out of those torture devices.

Men are no different. Their suits and outerwear can have padded shoulders to give "the look". Men don't tuck in their T-shirts because they think their bellies will be less noticeable that way. Men's foundation garments are making more visible appearances in mainstream menswear catalogs where formerly they were found hidden away in specialty publications. Men are having their flesh sliced open and risk reactions to anesthesia and improperly installed implants just to have these foreign objects slipped under their pecs and calves because they are too lazy to work out and build the real thing.

—And these implants *never* look like the real thing, for those who might be considering this, any more than the old doll-head hair plug transplants from the '70s and '80s looked like natural hair.

Both sexes are risking serious complications and death by having their flesh cut open and metal rods shoved brutally into their bodies to suck out fat. In 98% of all cases, fat will disappear with proper diet and a challenging fitness regimen. But of course, tens of millions claim exception because they've convinced themselves they're members of the hopeless 2% group.

The same people who dutifully maintain their cars, their homes and their relationships almost always fall short of maintaining their one and only irreplaceable body. And if your body fails, with it goes your ability to drive that car, maintain that house or maybe even hold onto that relationship.

We're Evaporating

If we are not intentionally building muscle after the age of 30, then we are continually, automatically losing muscle... up to 7% of our entire muscle mass per decade. How shocking is that?

That means a 50-year-old person has already lost fully 15% of their entire physical foundation, their level of strength, and their vigorous, vital appearance. A 70 year-old person has lost nearly a full third of the complete physical being they once were. This also means they've lost 30% of their ability to burn fat, as well as 30% of the power of their immune system to fight off illness and disease. And remember, your heart is a muscle too.

The most effective way for a woman or a man to turn back the hands of time is to rebuild the muscle they have lost through strength training, or even better, to build brand new muscle in key areas of their body where they never even had it before. This is how a man or woman can achieve a stronger and more attractive body after age 40 than they ever had in their younger days.

We can have our faces stretched and pulled and sculpted by the world's most talented plastic surgeons, but youth is a message broadcast by the entire body, not just the face. No surgeon can give you firm shapely muscle, impressive posture or the immeasurable level of self confidence that blossoms along with your body's transformation when that transformation is accomplished by your own hand.

When We Lose Muscle, We Are Literally Wasting Away.

When we lose muscle we are doing more than just getting smaller and weaker. We are eroding our immune system and providing disease a foothold. We are also diminishing our metabolism, the result of which is we become fatter without ever increasing our food intake.

Getting fat without the joy of eating our favorite foods? If that isn't most people's idea of hell, what is?

When we lose muscle, we are becoming physically more fragile and unsteady, and less attractive. Our sexual abilities and talents diminish as our muscle, and thus our strength, stamina and balance, ebbs. When muscle disappears, a woman's once shapely legs and the sexy back she used to proudly display in a swimsuit or backless dress disappear with it.

When muscle goes, a man's shoulders shrink and narrow, and the impressive arms of his youth wither. Loss of fat-burning muscle means the body accumulates more fat, especially in the belly. As our muscle fades away, our posture suffers as well, giving us a more bent and elderly appearance no matter what our actual chronological age, and bringing with it the onset of back problems.

Muscle symmetry and size in both women and men is what makes an attractive body attractive. Someone who stands straight and tall and exhibits exemplary muscle tone impresses everybody, whether via admiration or envy. If you match this particular physical description you are viewed as a stronger, kinder and more successful person whether or not in reality you are, or perhaps even as someone to be reckoned with.

It's becoming scientifically clear that our idea of beauty is not nearly the learned nor culturally-influenced behavior some would like us to believe it is. In one British experiment, six-month-old babies spent twice as much time studying images of the attractive faces they were shown on a TV monitor as they did unattractive ones. Obviously a six-month-old child has yet to be influenced by the media and so-called "unrealistic standards of beauty." Yet they were far more interested in, and intent on lingering upon, the more attractive faces.

Experiments done with 6 year olds in a US grade school revealed that between two unfamiliar substitute teachers allowed to temporarily lead their class, the more attractive teacher was perceived by the children to be smarter, stronger, nicer and more successful than the less attractive one. Interestingly, the two teachers were in fact the same person. In one guise she was dressed in a fat suit, fitted with fake crooked teeth, and unattractively groomed. In the other, she was "made over" to be at her prettiest.

Building and maintaining muscle must be a lifelong activity in order for us to function at optimum levels, both physically and psychologically, well into old age. Feeling strong and attractive, and *looking* strong and attractive, are the greatest gifts you could ever give yourself —and your loved ones. It's repeatedly said that people who are happy with themselves are more able and more likely to be giving to others than those embroiled in self-doubt.

Train at Home, Or At The Gym?

Many people would rather work out at home than at a gym for a number of reasons. It's certainly more convenient. At home there are no membership fees to pay, you don't have to worry about how you're dressed, and you don't have to wait around until someone finishes using the equipment that you want. There is no driving or public transportation involved, weather isn't a factor, you can work out in silence or to the music of your choice, and since no one is watching except the cat, you won't be self-conscious.

But there is a downside to working out at home as well: family interruptions, telephones, doorbells, food, favorite TV programs, the Internet and household chores, just to name just a few.

For successful results at home, you must aggressively claim workout time and space as your own. Your family and friends must accept the fact that you are not to be interrupted, and as difficult as this may sometimes be to enforce, you have to insist upon no exceptions to the rule.

Indeed, many people who are serious about their workouts end up joining a gym specifically just to get away from interruptions at home that they find impossible to control.

My main criticism of the workout articles and tutorials I see in fitness magazines and books is that the photos are too few and the written instruction is far too skimpy. Most workout routine articles picture just a "start" and "finish" photo, when so much *more* obviously goes on in between those two end points.

A major flaw in many magazine articles and videos is that the workout routines are not narrated by the professional who is pictured demonstrating the exercise, but instead are being described by an observer —or worse, a professional narrator with no workout experience.

No one can tell you how to perform an exercise like the qualified individual actually performing it. The ability to clearly explain what should be happening during the exercise is critical to getting the most bang for your buck. That is why the internet is such a boon. You can find hundreds of short videos online for free that feature trainers demonstrating the exercises. You can stop and start the videos, or watch certain parts over and over until you fully understand the technique.

You can make extraordinary progress working out at home by staying focused, and learning how to isolate each individual muscle or muscle group, which we call the target muscle. The greater your mental focus and concentration on the target muscle as it expands and contracts, the quicker and more impressive will be your physical progress.

Nothing will make us look younger or give the impression that we have reclaimed our youth more than regaining the precious muscle mass we have already lost, or even better, building brand new muscle in strategic areas where we've always wanted it but never had it before.

Weight Training Builds New Bone And Delays Aging

Weight training does more than make us stronger and improve our balance. Weight training builds bone —brand new strong bone. Taking calcium or a prescription drug like *Fosamax* (which as of this writing has been found to have some serious side effects) are two treatments many use in their attempt to avoid osteoporosis, but weight training is far and away exceedingly superior. Strength training is the only known way to actually build entirely new bone.

You may already be aware that one of the first things that scientists noticed about astronauts returning to earth was bone loss. This bone loss was directly due to physical inactivity and the lack of stress placed on bone in a weightless environment. Scientific measurement taken in studies of people who use one hand or one arm more than the other for heavy work, specifically tennis players and lumberjacks, showed the bones in the active arm and hands were significantly larger than in the less active arm.

I had worked out with weights pretty consistently from age 12 until age 34. Then, frustrated with not looking the way I had always wanted to look, I began working out with a talented competitive bodybuilder named Mike Hage. He was the same height as I was, and we had the same waist size, yet he weighed 50 lbs. more than I did, and that 50 lbs. was all muscle. This workout experience with him changed my life, because I had always convinced myself that I was a hard worker at the gym. I soon learned that my new partner was upping the ante and I was astonished at the increase in effort and energy that was required for me to keep up with him. I had to drink a lot more water, sleep more, and eat more of the right kinds of food to fuel the workouts and optimize my results. But I also quickly acclimated to this increased demand on my body, and within 6 weeks I not only looked dramatically different, but could keep up the pace right along with Mike.

I was very happy to see my muscles growing, but I was really surprised to see that my hands and wrists were growing in size as well. Firmly gripping heavy weights day in and day out for a year increased my hand size noticeably, a benefit that was totally unexpected. I had always had small hands and wrists, and in the beginning of my new program back then, they seemed to be my weak link, as gripping heavy weights made them cramp up, but soon both were growing in size along with the rest of my muscles.

Aren't I Too Old To Recreate My Body, Much Less Build Brand-New Muscle And Bone?

When I was in college at age 19, I had a classmate who was 29 and in bad physical shape. I urged him to do something about it after tiring of hearing him complain about how unhappy he was with the way he looked and how fatigued he felt all the time. But his response was "Its too late for me…I'm 29! When you get to be my age you can't change your body that way anymore." Even back then with my limited experience and knowledge about physical fitness his statement took me aback, because he didn't seem like he was just making excuses. That poor guy really believed, at only age 29, that he was too old to change his body.

In studies involving both male and female residents of retirement homes conducted in the US and Great Britain, science has proven that well into our 90s humans have the ability to build substantial lean muscle mass through strength training. Physiologically, we are all programmed to live to be older than 100 years, and at no time are we incapable of building bigger, stronger muscles.

There are presently more than 70,000 people over the age of 100 living in the United States, and by my own one hundredth birthday in 2049, it is projected that there will be over a million. As baseball great Mickey Mantle once said, "If I knew I was going to live this long, I would have taken a whole lot better care of myself".

Illness may not be something we can successfully avoid, but physical weakness is preventable. The aches and pains, stumbling and falling, lack of energy and lethargy that are attributed to "getting older" all stem from physical weakness, *not from aging itself.*

The need to become physically stronger actually increases with age, yet in reality, few people ever strive to become physically stronger as they get older.

Why is this? Why have we embraced the irrational idea that, just as we start to become physically weaker, we need to slow down?

If we become sick, our intuition and survival instinct *should* prompt us to do those things that will make us well again. When we're tired, we sleep to recharge our energy cells. When we're hungry we eat. But for most people, the signs that they are diminishing physically does not prompt the rational response of engaging in activities that will make them stronger, whether it be rehabilitation for an injury, or exercise. Even stranger, people with chromic injuries, such as a foot, knee or shoulder injury that impedes their every movement, do not seek out physical therapy. A quality physical therapist is your gold standard when it comes to fixing your physical problems. My good friend's mother, who was very well off financially and liked me quite a bit, would not even let me talk to her about seeing a physical therapist to attend to her badly injured knee. For months she limped around, the pain quite obvious, and it became worse as time went on, yet she never sought treatment. It's bad enough when a 20 year old thinks he's invincible, and believes his injury will get better all by itself. But when a senior plows on despite severely compromised mobility, and refuses treatment? Well, that's a mental problem, not just a physical one.

Even though the ability to add muscle and bone, strengthen

joints and increase endurance never diminishes with age, it is true that, due to a lifetime of wear and tear and a loss of elasticity, older bodies are somewhat more susceptible to injury, be it related to household chores, gardening, or exercise. A physical therapist can help you regain lost mobility, and give you your life back.

When strength training, jogging, or using a cardio machine like a treadmill or stair stepper, keeping our minds fully engaged during the actual exercise is the best way to avoid injury. Lots of people pass the tedium of walking on a treadmill by watching TV. Make sure that if you do this, you do not zone out on the TV and completely disengage from the primary task at hand. There are tens of thousands of treadmill injuries annually, most due to inattentiveness. Even ultra-fit singer Madonna suffered one such injury in 2009. It may seem like a mindless endeavor, but walking or running on a treadmill does require your attention.

The US Consumer Products Safety Commission reports that in a recent average year, 90,000 Americans ended up in the hospital due to accidents involving gardening equipment alone. One's home environment has proven far more dangerous than any gym, but the reason for accidents and injuries in both places is the same.

This same philosophy must be applied whenever you exercise, no matter what exercise you choose. Your mind cannot wander, nor can you be trying to watch TV (unless you are following instructions on a video) or read at the same time you are strength training. Not having one's mind fully engaged in the exercise is the number one cause of exercise-related injury.

So it is doubly important that we think before we do, and mentally divide each exercise into controlled segments. Just jumping on an exercise machine without fully knowing how to use it and going at it full throttle like we're on some ride at Disneyland isn't even a good idea for a 20 year old, much less someone over 40.

I witness people of all ages at the gym slamming the too-heavy weight stacks and thrashing around spastically on machines, the machine being in control of them, rather than vice-versa. Which brings to mind those gym-goers who invent their own exercises, usually resembling someone in the throes of an epileptic seizure.

I was born in 1949, and except for mild scoliosis, an irregular curvature of the spine, there is nothing really unusual about my physicality. I am naturally an ectomorph, with slim bones and small joints. At my full height [just under 5'9"] at age 21 I weighed 125 lbs. The reason I want people to know this is so that they will not think that I am a "naturally big guy" who started out with a physical advantage others don't have. I have intentionally built every ounce of muscle over and above the 125 lbs. that I began with as an adult.

I am a little embarrassed to admit it, but although I have always weight trained, I was not inspired to tackle a truly solid and focused training and nutrition plan that excelled for me until I was in my mid-40s. I made better muscle gains between the ages of 46 and 50 than at any other time of my life. At age 46 I weighed 158 lbs. At age 50 I weighed 185 lbs., with 7% body fat. I had gained 23 lbs. of muscle and bone between the ages of 18 and 46, a span of almost 30 years. I gained 27 lbs. of muscle and bone between the ages of 46 and 50, a span of four years, at a time in life lyrically known as "over the hill".

In my experience I have encountered people who, as they speak with me, seem to be taking mental notes and reassessing their lifestyle. There are relatively few people over 50 in acceptable physical shape, much less in excellent shape. Just realizing that someone their own age who is just as just busy as they are has "done it" is sometimes enough to convince some that it is not too late to make a change.

For those in a big hurry to reverse years of bad decisions, keep in mind that you can't undo decades of damage and abuse in just a few weeks. It took years for you to get into bad shape, so it will take time, but much less time to be sure, to whip yourself into great shape.

With strength training you can make noticeable changes in the way you look and feel in 4 weeks. Soon people will be commenting on the transformation taking place, something that will most certainly encourage you to keep moving forward. But you can never think of this change in your routine as temporary. Like brushing your teeth, strength training and improved diet must be adopted as ongoing habit. You cannot think that you can strength train and eat intelligently for the next 90 days, and then continue to hold on to the new improved you if you revert back to your former ways.

People like to say. "I lost the fat, but it came back." *Lost fat never comes back*. When you lose fat, that fat is gone forever. If you get fat *again*, that fat is brand-new fat, newly created and nurtured by your most recent lifestyle choices.

Also, muscle does not change to fat, turn into fat, or vice versa, any more than apples turn into oranges. Muscle and fat are completely different, non-interchangeable things.

If we want to keep our teeth, we'll brush and floss every day. If we want to keep our youth, we'll be just as faithful to our ongoing strength training schedule and a sound nutritional program.

Time and aging do take a toll, and nothing invented so far will give us back the taut and elastic skin we had in our youth. For those of you who are not excessively overweight, adding muscle, even in small amounts, will "fill up" the loose skin, making it appear tighter...and indeed it will be, because you've created more flesh beneath it to enclose.

Those who were once overweight, or want to lose weight should realistically know that your skin may not contract as much as you'd like as you lose weight, depending on your genetics, because its elasticity is limited. But since we spend most of our waking hours with clothes on, this may be a minor point for you.

Without exaggeration, by age 55 I had achieved a better developed, better looking, stronger and harder body than any previous year in my entire life. Although you may have the desire to achieve results that are unique to your own vision, it is undeniable that in addition to the health, strength and mobility benefits, you will create a more attractive body when you strength train and eat nutritionally sound foods.

I was able to lift heavier weights, more safely, in my 50s than at any previous time in my life. In recent years my knees had been exhibiting classic aging signs, due in part to having small joints and employing less than perfect technique while weight training when I was younger. In having to relearn how to work my legs in order to avoid this knee pain, I discovered, and corrected, that which I had previously been doing that exacerbated the problem: I had been driving my leg exercises from my knees, instead of from my glutes, or rear end. During squats, leg presses, lunges, or just climbing stairs, I was propelling myself and absorbing the shock with my knees, rather than powering up, and putting the breaks on, using my glutes.

So as I encourage you to strength train, I can, with the benefit of 30 years of serious weight training, personal training and the successes and mistakes accumulated over the years, steer you away from the unwise, the unproductive and the injurious. A testament to my learning from my own mistakes, fixing them, and being able to offer advice and counsel, is that at nearly sixty years of age, I stand alone in almost any gym I walk into, from New York to Honolulu. The reason why there are so few men my age who have the kind of physique I have, and feel the way I do, is because as younger less careful men, others ate, injured or simply used themselves up.

Whatever your goals, from modest to extravagant, be assured that you can achieve practically anything you put your mind to. And unlike a wildly successful career or world-wide fame or other goals people have set for themselves, you need nobody's cooperation or permission to achieve greatness here.

You do not have to wait around until "someday" for it to happen, or for things to finally go your way. You begin today, make it part of your day-to-day regimen like all the other regimens you've already taken on, and your success will become visible in two weeks, and will continue and expand from that day forward. We all have 24 hours in our day, and we all decide how to fill them. Learn to say "no" to those things that do not enhance your life, and "yes" to those that do.

Whether you have never worked out with weights in your life, or you are beginning again after a layoff period, you must begin slowly. Besides following the instruction in this book, allow common sense to guide you along your path of accomplishment. It is natural for us as human beings to want what we want as soon as possible. But keep in mind that the next year is going to pass regardless, and "steady as she goes" will get you to an impressive place faster and safer than any mad rush.

Don't Get Discouraged By Setbacks

Setbacks are a fact of life. Life's events get in the way, and they must be accommodated. My muscle weight fluctuates by 20 pounds or more, depending on multiple factors. When I live far from the gym rather than close, when I need to work longer hours to make ends meet, when the only gym available is very poorly maintained and equipped, when a loved one becomes ill —all those things and more take attention and time away from my strength training goals. But at no time do I ever completely stop eating right or stop going to the gym. At times I have only been able to work out once every ten days, and as I looked in the mirror and saw the loss of my hard-won gains, as discouraging as that was, I knew the hard times would end, as they always have, and then I would win back what I had lost.

And by staying in the game, even if it sometimes was at a much reduced level, I was always poised to go at it again full steam when circumstances improved.

Should I Consult My Doctor First?

You should if you have been sedentary for a long time, or if you haven't seen a doctor within the last year. I'm one of those more unusual people who is not afraid to visit the doctor, probably because I always expect good news, and usually get it. If a problem is revealed, I do whatever it takes to fix it. Those who fear the prospect of bad news…well, that fear alone should tell you it's time for your check up.

Both of my older brothers, who are three years apart in age, had their first heart attacks at age 38. My dad died from his first heart attack, at age 46. So when I decided to team up with bodybuilder Mike Hage at age 34 and allow myself to be pushed to my limits, I needed to feel I was beginning this journey safely. Although my lifestyle was the polar opposite of my brothers', I still wanted a professional assessment.

I know that a healthy lifestyle can overcome bad genetics, and the proof of that was revealed by the excellent results of my electrocardiogram and stress tests. But at age 60, I had still never experienced any heart problems, even though my older brothers both had in their 30s. My younger brother too quit smoking and took up marathon racing at age 29, and at age 52 is still running, and still very healthy.

Can I Really Sculpt My Body?

Yes. You not only can change the shape of your body as a whole, but you can add size to any given muscle or muscle group to bring it up to par with the rest of your body. We call this creating symmetry. For example, you can visually minimize a genetically predetermined wide waist by increasing the size of your shoulders and the width of your back. Instead of ladies relying on shoulder pads to give them the look they are after, they can increase the size of their shoulders for real. People who have a saggy butt, or no butt, can build an impressive amount of muscle in this area and completely transform this body part.

Women should not be afraid that they are going to acquire the look of a professional female bodybuilder. The pumped-up freaky gaunt-faced look that some female bodybuilders aspire to is overwhelmingly the result of *extreme* administration of male hormones in the form of steroids or testosterone —even though most deny the dead-obvious. To which I reply, the gyms of the world are filled with men who struggle to build muscles half as big as those which some female bodybuilders have, and yet those men have ample amounts of naturally-occurring testosterone coursing through their veins. And these women want you to believe that they who produce virtually no testosterone are able to create massive male-like bodies without it?

Genetically, without chemical manipulation, females simply cannot look like this, and neither can you. Besides, the down side about building muscle is that if we stop, most of the new muscle we've built disappears over time. *If we're not actively building muscle, we're actively losing muscle.*

Unlike the myth of spot reduction, in which people erroneously believe they can reduce the amount of fat in a certain body part without affecting the rest of the body, body-sculpting via strength training is very real. You can add size to your shoulders, or your forearms, your calves or virtually any other body part while having relatively minor effect on other muscles, by isolating the target muscle.

Adding size to certain body parts will make other troublesome body parts appear smaller. And the fat burning effects of weight training will remove fat from problem areas such as thighs, waist and stomach, but in a uniform manner. However, you cannot diminish the size of a chosen muscle, or lessen the size of bones or joints.

Women who have "cottage cheese" thighs or butt will be pleased to know that weight training exercises coupled with a healthful nutritional plan can give their thighs a lean, smooth look. With weight training, you really can turn back the clock.

Actually, as you become proficient in strength training and you begin to see the results, you will realize that the idea of weight training solely to remodel a single body part was naive, because you will realize how all the muscles work in tandem to create an ideal look. Nobody would disagree that big arms hanging from little shoulders just looks silly.

Once you observe the first changes in your physique, you will gain a greater appreciation as to how all the muscles tie together, how they work together to form a complete look. Strength training will make you much more body-aware, of yourself, and others.

We reside in our bodies 24 hours a day and carry them everywhere we go, yet most people don't know the first thing about theirs. People who do not engage in physical activity are disturbingly unaware of their anatomy, what it looks like and how it all works, how they hold themselves, how vital it is to take care of their one and only body, and most important, how crucial it is to use and move theirs correctly.

The majority of people whose bodies "are failing them" are in truth people who have failed their bodies. One cannot expect to spend a lifetime ignoring, misusing and abusing one's body and not end up paying a heavy price.

Just Picture Yourself...

If you have a realistic picture of yourself, you probably already have some idea of what your body's strong and weak points are. You may already know that you would be more pleased with your look if your legs weren't as skinny, or if your shoulders were larger.

I cannot stress strongly enough the benefit of taking photos of yourself, both at the beginning of your program, and monthly as you progress. If you are like most people, others will notice a change in your appearance even before you do. Looking at ourselves many times a day, the changes may seem almost imperceptible, but to those who have not seen us in a few weeks, the changes will be much more pronounced. And seeing your progress in a photo is far more revealing than just looking at yourself in a mirror.

If you have a self-timing device on your camera, you can take the photos yourself by placing the camera on a tripod or table. If not, ask a friend or relative to take the shots. Pose the same way each time, in a bathing suit. The photo should be taken in the same place with the same light source each time. You want the lighting and location to be the same every time because these two factors can make a big difference in the way your body appears in photos.

If you study the before and after photos used in ads for things like wrinkle creams, you will often see that very unflattering, hard lighting was used for the "before" shot. For the "after shot", softer more flattering lighting was used to enhance the illusion of improvement, or sometimes to photographically create results that aren't even real. For progress shots, you want a *true picture* of your development rather than the most flattering picture of yourself.

These photos that you take, placed side by side as you progress, will probably amaze you. It is difficult to convince people of just what they are capable of accomplishing until they view graphic proof for themselves.

Strength training is work. No one can deny that. But I believe you will be surprised that it is not as hard as you thought it would be, and that the results will come faster than you imagined they would, especially if you change your diet so that the bulk of what you eat contributes to growing a healthy, attractive body.

Compare Yourself

Because women especially have bought into the popular "unrealistic standards of beauty" nonsense, they have allowed their options to diminish by doing so. Anyone who has such low self esteem that they feel personally diminished simply by looking at a photo of a beautiful person in a magazine needs to do as much work at the psychotherapist's office as they do in the gym.

A high school swimmer who dreams of greatness will not strive to be more like the guy in the next lane, but in most cases will choose a hero of Olympic stature. Makes sense. We all need something to aim for, even if we don't think we have a realistic chance of fully reaching our fantasy goal. We all need role models.
Similarly, whether male or female, you should choose a role model whose physique you admire and whose achievements will inspire you to keep moving forward and improving.

Looking at yourself in the mirror will not reveal your progress fully, nor your weak areas that need improvement. Posing for a photo in your swimsuit in the same pose as one of your role models, and studying them side-by-side, will quickly reveal what parts of your body need primary attention.

Until my 40s, I was unaware of how proportionately small my shoulders were until I copied a pose of one of my role models and compared my photos side-by-side with his. Immediately what I was lacking jumped right out at me. How had I not seen that before?

Indeed there were other discrepancies as well, but it was the deltoid difference that really surprised me. Beginning that same day, shoulders became my new priority at the gym, and have continued to be.

At another gym I belonged to when I was 52, there was a 20-year-old kid with movie star looks and contest-quality physique who strutted around the place like he was God's gift to planet earth. His saving grace was that he was very friendly, complimentary and respectful.

After a few instances of him complimenting me, one afternoon when the gym was almost empty I walked past him and his workout partner as they rested between sets, and he laughed at me and mocked, "When are you gonna start working on those pencil forearms? They look lame hanging from those big biceps!"

He had set me up with compliments, then hit me with a zinger, which, as I studied my arms in the mirror, I had to conclude was dead on.

How did I not notice before, with all my work and hard-won gains, that I had comparatively underdeveloped forearms? When I went home I took out my progress pictures and compared them to my role model, and yikes, there it was. I had minor muscle size in my forearms, especially when compared to all my other gains. Pretty Boy was right.

Maybe some people can assess their progress just by looking in the mirror at the gym, but apparently I wasn't one of them. From then on, progress photos and comparisons with my role models has been an important part of my routine.

Women and Weight Training

I was very impressed by a town meeting I attended at the 92nd St. Y in New York City, where the late Governor Ann Richards [D-Texas, 1990-1995], a highly intelligent and very sought-after speaker, was asked about her signature Texas Big Hair. She drawled, "My hairdresser says you gotta have big hair to distract from a big rear end. It's all a matter of scale."

Among a host of other topics, she spoke eloquently about the impact that her mother's death had had on her. She said she had watched her elderly mother break into "bits and pieces" as she fractured bone after bone due to osteoporosis. Frightened by witnessing her mother's plight, and fearing that she too had this disease, Gov. Richards went to her doctor for a bone density scan. She found that she was in the early stages of the disease. She had thought that there was nothing she could do. She said that she believed she would end up with a neck one inch long and stooped over, with a big hump on her back. That is, until she learned about strength training.

Her response was to immediately begin weight training, for the first time in her life. She was then in her 60s.

She stated correctly that weight training is the only way a woman (or a man) can add actual bone density and growth, and she not only felt great, but by her own admission looked "fabulous". No argument there.

Governor Richards went on to describe herself as the world's most public alcoholic, sober since 1980. Anyone who has read about the amazing life she led would probably agree that after all the trauma, upheaval and joy she experienced that she had finally earned the right to do nothing but sit around and watch TV all day in restful retirement.

Instead she decided to go to work as a lobbyist in Washington DC, and make the rounds on the lecture circuit, traveling all over the US. In her "spare" time keeping an eye on her children and 7 grandchildren. Yet, despite a schedule that would cripple a 25 year old, she *made*, not "found", the time to weight train religiously. Described by fans and critics alike as never one to surrender, Governor Richards was determined that osteoporosis would not conquer her, but with the help of weight training, she would conquer osteoporosis.

In another example, actress Debbie Reynolds was incredulous in an interview that with her documented family history of osteoporosis —both her mother and grandmother suffered from it— that her primary care physician never suggested a bone density scan. It was not until she first heard about the availability of bone density scans that she confronted her doctor about it. Subsequently, she found that indeed she was well along in the progression of osteoporosis upon receiving the results of the scan. This is a great example of how you can be world famous, well off financially, and have access to all the best doctors, and still not have your health properly attended to.

It is recommended that all women over the age of 40 have a bone density scan. Osteoporosis can do major damage before it is detected, and like most diseases, is more successfully treated in its earliest stages.

Weight training will build and strengthen and create brand-new bone. The earlier the disease is diagnosed, the more easily it can be arrested.

Out Of Shape

Interestingly, the more out of shape you are, the more dramatic your progress will be. The older you are, the more striking will be your transformation as well. We're mildly impressed when an out-of-shape 30 year old reinvents their physique. But when a 50 year old does it? People *really* sit up and take notice.

In yet another Tufts University study involving 90-year-old women and regular strength training, the average woman in this study increased her muscle mass by 9%, and her actual physical strength by a whopping 100% in only twelve weeks.

Chapter 4
The Open Secrets Of Strength Training

The secret to quick results and injury-free strength training is flexing.

My workout partner Alex del Rosario MD and I shot videos of our workouts to monitor our form and progress. I had planned on doing an instructional DVD for quite a while, but when I reviewed these tapes, I found they looked far better than I'd realized and demonstrated exactly what I wanted to teach people. Videographers who shoot bodybuilding and fitness videos are rarely bodybuilders themselves, so they don't have a very good handle on what to zero in on as they film: *we do*.

My DVD is not a super-polished Hollywood studio/MTV-style music video like so many I have seen. Those videos might look snazzy, but the fast editing cuts and other effects are distractions that diminish the educational value of the instruction, and ultimately leave me feeling disappointed due to their lack of substance. In my DVD I describe exactly and in great detail what we are doing, and why. But most importantly I tell you, the viewer, what you should be *doing and feeling*.

95% of the people I see in the gym are doing their exercises wrong, or at best, ineffectively. The principals outlined in my chosen exercises on my DVD are meant to be applied across the board, no matter what exercises you choose for your own routine, whether they be the same as mine or from another source. The underlying principals are always the same, no matter what muscle group you are working, and no matter which exercise you are performing.

It isn't what you do, or how much weight you use, it's how you perform the exercises that quickly strengthens and builds muscle.

You can find my **WORKOUT PhD** DVD and free sample clips at <www.discoveringhawaii.com>. Click on the *Fitness* link at the top of the page.

Introduction To Strength Training

Just ahead of you await a new body, unaccustomed strength, a better sex life, less depression, a stronger immune system, and increased fat-burning capability and energy. Strength training is nothing to be afraid of, unless you have a fear of shopping for new clothes, or getting a lot more involved in living a vibrant life.

How to Work Out With Weights

It's not so much what you do, it's how you do it. There are really no new exercises; there are just new ways to go about performing the tried-and-true ones. And *flexing* is the key.

You can work out —with weights, Pilates, aerobics, whatever— either with full focus and flawless technique, or in a lazy, lackadaisical, haphazard way. Whatever your choice, you'll get out of it exactly what you put into it.

Approach your workout with focus, drive, and a vivid picture of your goal in mind, and you will accomplish much. Approach your workout grudgingly, as if it's some horrible chore you are being forced into and just can't wait to finish, and you will accomplish far less. Yet, the time invested for either result is exactly the same. Performing exercises slowly & deliberately with focused concentration will bring life-altering results and keep you safe from injury.

Actors in the acclaimed TV series *Mad Men,* which is set in the early 1960s, talk about how crucially the wardrobe contributes to their performance. The men say their tight skinny suits compel them to stand up straight and put them in a totally different state of mind. The actresses' girdles and foundation garments remind them at all times they are indeed in a different era. Their characters stand and walk differently than the actors themselves do.

Choose wardrobe for your workout that will put you in the proper frame of mind. You need to see your muscles in motion, so at least wear something that reveals the current body part you are working on. If today you want to work arms, wear a tank top or a sleeveless shirt, for example. Maybe you wouldn't be caught dead wearing spandex in public, but if working out at home in spandex gets you in the right frame of mind, then go for it.

Gerard Butler, who starred in the eye-boggling film *300,* and who ordinarily does not work out, trained for up to six hours a day for his role as King Lionedes. Not only did he have to train just like a bodybuilder to attain the physique required of the character, but also had rigorous swordplay, shield and spear training, as well as boot camp instruction to maximize his agility and stamina. His physical training for the role spanned a full year.

In his interviews he lights up when explaining how crucial this physical training was to his ability to fully inhabit the role in which he was cast. He explains that before shooting each scene he pumped up with weights that were kept close at hand. He didn't have to "act" like an awesomely built warrior, because he had in reality *become one.*

"When you do a scene right after you've just finished pumping up, you feel amazing, physically, but you also feel the fire burning inside without you having to fake it. And therefore the huge value from (getting pumped-up) was ... acting preparation. So I used that preparation the whole way through the shoot. If you can focus the entire time on being all-powerful, then you are all-powerful. If you believe it, you are."

Gerry had a goal, a purpose, an end-date, and tremendous motivation: career, salary, maintaining his reputation for giving his all, and the knowledge that he will live on gloriously in this on-screen presence no matter what the future brings.

You and I have more modest reasons and goals —millions of people will not be sitting in theaters around the world watching us in awe on the big screen, but the personal payoff for us may be no less significant than Gerry's was for him.

It is impossible to describe the intense feeling of power and confidence that comes from taking control of your own being and your own destiny, and transforming your own physique and health for the better.

The most important piece of equipment that we can bring to our workout is the *right attitude*: enthusiasm, optimism, commitment, a vivid mind-picture of how we want to look to ourselves and to others, how we want to feel, both short-term and long-term goals, and the mind-set of "If you believe it, you *are*".

The Wrong Way

Remember *GIGO:* it means garbage in, garbage out. We get out of our workout exactly what we put into it.

After 40 years in gyms I can safely say that the majority of men and women in any gym at any given moment have poor workout technique: they perform the exercises incorrectly, with poor form and lack of focus and commitment, and therefore attain minor progress. Even when watching world-class personal trainer Charles Glass in his bodybuilding.com video series, it was interesting to see people in the background of the shot at Gold's Gym Venice utilizing such poor technique. There they are working out in the most famous gym in the world, surrounded by some of the planet's most awesome physiques, and it doesn't occur to them to watch, learn, and mimic the technique of these champions?

After setting aside time for the workout, getting dressed for it, driving to the gym, paying your gym membership, etc., it makes no sense to then spend your workout time socializing or daydreaming. If you are going to commit to your workout, it makes no sense *not* to be researching, *not* to be reading bodybuilding and fitness magazines, watching video instruction, learning, and emulating role models.

Don't Just Spin Your Wheels

I've observed all kinds of odd behavior at the gym, but the most common is avoidance: people spend the entire time talking, daydreaming, watching the TV monitors. They pay their membership dues, show up at the gym, then slack off.

One person I am thinking of made no progress in four years. He keeps a clip board at one location in the gym, performs an unchallenging set of whatever exercise, immediately gets up from the machine, walks clear across the gym, and notes something on the clip board, walks back across the gym and does another mediocre set. Then, he gets up, and repeats the odd ritual. He could keep the clip board with him, eliminating the need to walk across the gym dozens of times. He could wait until the end of the exercise to make his notes, but all this walking around and busy work allows him to keep up his pretense. He likes to turn on the TV, play a DVD of some massive bodybuilder taking viewers through his championship routine, turning the volume up loud, yet obviously does not follow any of the bodybuilder's advice. He is filling up all his workout time with unproductive busy work and distractions in order to avoid doing any real work. In his head he's probably fooled himself into believing he's committed, present, and enthused. Yet, in four years, he has not made any transformation for the better whatsoever. He rarely challenges himself physically, has made no changes to his diet (after 4 years he still had a belly), nor has he ever pushed himself far enough beyond his present routine so that positive change in his physique would be visible.

At the opposite end of the spectrum, there was a very overweight little 13 year old Armenian boy who joined the gym, who I paid little attention to until one day I was delighted to notice he wasn't fat anymore. Within less than a year he had transformed from a roly-poly child who looked about 12, to a 14 year old buffed young man who looked closer to 16. I admired his commitment and drive at such a young age, but then I *really* admired him when he marched up to me one day and announced that I was his "hero", and that watching me workout "and not talk to anybody" was his inspiration. I knew that I would never have had the courage to approach someone like me when I was his age, especially someone who didn't "talk to anybody". I congratulated him sincerely on what he had accomplished thus far, and told him that the sky was the limit for someone with his personality, focus and healthy self-esteem. He beamed because someone he admired told him he was admired as well. I recalled what that felt like, when I was his age, to have someone I looked up to praise and encourage me…it meant everything.

Just Do It… Right.

The reason why people hurt themselves while pursuing any fitness activity, like jogging, aerobics or strength training, is because they're not doing it right. "Doing it right" is a combination of accepting the instruction of someone who has already mastered the activity, remaining focused on the immediate task at hand, and paying attention to your own gut feelings.

Feeling discomfort is part of the process. Feeling pain is not.

Imagine going for a jog wearing a backpack with three or four bricks in it. That's what jogging is like for an overweight person, and adjustments in the way overweight individuals exercise must be made to accommodate the excess weight throwing them off balance until it's lost. Muscles get stronger with use, but joints do not…they wear out. Excess weight especially places a lot of stress on knees and lower back during exercise. Begin slowly, stay focused and move deliberately.

Overweight beginners should place their major emphasis at first on developing core strength by concentrating on *unweighted* abdominal, lower back and intercostals (the muscles along the sides of your torso) exercises, while at the same time making changes in their diet. There are a few adjustments you can make while performing exercises to guard your lower back. When lying on your back on a bench to do chest exercises, for example, bend your legs at the knees and keep your feet up on the bench rather than placing them flat on the floor. This will keep you from arching your back, which would place more negative stress on it. Avoid arching your back no matter what the exercise.

When standing to perform biceps curls or front or lateral raises for the shoulder, try keeping your back flush against a wall, tilting your pelvis slightly to press the lumbar vertebrae into the wall as you raise and lower the weight in a focused fashion.

Geezercise

The most significant limitations older people have when it comes to strength training are those related to wear and tear. Some twenty-year-olds may have already suffered significant wear and tear, while some seventy year olds have relatively little. It depends, among other things, on what physical demands have been placed on your body, and how self-aware you were when you performed physical tasks in your past.

Any health problems must be considered, but the truth is that far more people have heart attacks sitting around doing nothing than do those who strength train, so your doctor will be your best guide.

Your Best Allies: A Sports Medicine Doctor And A Physical Therapist

Those with existing medical conditions who are determined to strength train will find their best ally and guide in a sports medicine doctor working in conjunction with the medical specialist treating their primary problem. If there's a way to get you active again, the sports med doc will be the one to know. He will work in collaboration with your specialist and/or physical therapist to devise a workout regime that will keep you safe while at the same time insuring results. To locate the best sports medicine physician in your area, contact the local university and ask who treats their athletic teams.

The Engine

If you have never weight trained before, or haven't in years, begin slowly and deliberately. Power up using the target muscle itself to propel the weight throughout the exercise, rather than driving the exercise with your hands.

The object is not to lift the weight by raising your hand, despite the misleading term "weight lifting". The object is to contract, or flex, the target muscle forcefully, which in turn will drive the weight into motion.

There's a major difference between pushing or pulling a weight with your hands, and contracting/flexing the target muscle to propel the weight into motion.

Your hands have little to do with any exercise...all they do is attach you to the weight. Your hands are merely handles.

The engine that drives any given exercise is housed within the target muscle.

The Target Muscle

The muscle that any given exercise is designed to isolate and challenge is called the *target muscle.*

Most people propel each exercise primarily with their hands and focus on their hand, the dumbbell, or pulley handle: *this is wrong.*

Your hands are simply attachments, handles that connect you to the weight.

The weight is merely the object that provides the resistance for your target muscle to resist.

It is your target muscle that needs your full attention, not the weight, and not your hands.

You move the weight by first flexing/contracting the target muscle, and then powering up from the target muscle, rather than powering up from your hand.

When doing shoulder upright rows (which can be performed with a barbell, dumbbells, cable or specialized machine), for example,

I often overhear trainers telling their clients to raise their elbows higher in an attempt, I assume, to get them to perform the exercise more fruitfully. In reality, you need to get into position, flex your shoulders immediately before beginning the movement, and drive the weight up by engaging the engine located within your shoulders, not by involving your elbows. The flex in your shoulder at the apex of the exercise will determine "how high" the weight goes.

"How high" is *not* the goal. The goal is *not* to hoist the weight as high as possible. The goal is to propel the weight within its natural trajectory by forcefully flexing and contracting the shoulder muscles: your elbows, or hands, should never be the primary focus.

Your hands and elbows have nothing to do with raising the weight during shoulder exercises: the shoulders raise the weight during shoulder exercises, by the action of their contracting/flexing.

Your hands and surrounding muscles *can* raise the weight higher than the natural limit of your shoulders' flexing, but to so do you would have to disengage the shoulder muscles, defeating the purpose. Your shoulders drive all shoulder exercises, not your hands or elbows. Allow your hands to simply follow your flexing shoulder muscles' lead, not the other way around.

Keeping the target muscle, in this case the shoulders, flexed throughout the entire set of repetitions will provide the safest exercise form, and the most rewarding results. Relaxing, or letting go of the flex, or contraction, with every rep, as most people tend to do, allows the target muscle to disengage from the arc you've set, and the muscle is therefore less challenged, accomplishes less, and becomes more vulnerable to injury.

Consider The Whole Picture.

Nothing will benefit a person more universally than strength training, because nothing else compares in its ability to increase physical strength and function so dramatically.

Those individuals who consistently ignore training certain parts of their body, such as legs or back, end up looking off-kilter. They also leave themselves vulnerable by increasing the strength and stamina of one area of their body while leaving another comparatively weaker and unbalanced.

Very commonly, males tend to work at creating a buffed upper body while ignoring their legs. Their concealment strategy is to wear long pants at the gym. Many females often have little idea as to how to create a balanced look and uniform strength as well. This is not a criticism, for we all tend to focus on what we believe is our major flaw or strength, not realizing how blind we are to other problem areas we may also have.

When strength training you will find you have favorite body parts. If your arms develop quickly you'll most likely favor them and look forward to working them, because we are by nature driven and inspired by our successes. If working legs is less rewarding or more physically taxing than working arms, you'll be tempted to cut the leg workout short, or perform the leg exercises in a less than committed fashion. Stay focused and give all body parts equal attention to avoid weak areas and an unbalanced look.

More often than not you will find that the body parts you once hated working on soon become your favorites upon seeing them blossom.

When you begin to see how your newly toned and shaped hamstrings tie in with and compliment your recently firmed up rear end, you'll understand why you've been working a muscle you rarely get see for yourself in the mirror (but that everybody else sees), and you'll have that "ah-ha!" moment of understanding about how it all ties together to work as a unified whole. People have a tendency to blow off the exercises for muscles they can't see in the mirror, like hamstrings, or back.

Equipment: No Milk Jugs, Ever

When I see some air-headed "instructor" on some TV morning show tell people they can use plastic milk jugs, loaded grocery bags or even their baby (!) to exercise with, my blood pressure shoots up. Balance is the key to avoiding injury and a milk jug or loaded grocery bag will injure you quicker than it could ever benefit you, and only a true dumbbell would ever consider using a human child as ballast. So reject that kind of cockeyed advice.

Dumbbells are relatively inexpensive and available at all the big box stores like Costco and Wal-Mart, and very commonly at garage sales and on craigslist.com. The fixed-weight models are a better choice as opposed to the ones with interchangeable plates. The exposed ends of the bars on the interchangeable plate models will get in your way and can give you some nasty bruises to boot. And you don't want a weight plate accidentally slipping off the bar and breaking your toes. But in the end, work with what you can get or what's most comfortable for you.

It's understandable that people don't want to have a workout bench sitting in their living room, but when it's cleverly disguised as an ottoman, your workout bench becomes an attractive piece of furniture. I had mine built at a local upholstery shop and is slip covered for easy washing. I also cover the slipcover with a large beach towel when I use it for my workout. I had it built firmly for secure support and so that it does not move or wobble while I exercise. It may be possible to find an appropriate-sized ottoman at a second hand store. Ideally it should be 36 inches long or longer and about 24 inches wide. The ideal height is relational to your own height and the ease in allowing you to get up from a reclining position. Try a few on for size at the local furniture store before committing.

At home you will need a mirror, the bigger the better. Full-length is best.

A home chin-up/pull-up bar that spans a doorway is a great and inexpensive investment. Do not be tempted to install it without the support braces that firmly screw into the door frame. Test it before committing it to your full weight by keeping your feet on a secure stool that will partially support your weight. Besides pull-ups being an excellent overall upper body exercise, it feels great just to hang and stretch for a minute as you pass by the bar during the day. If you have a workout space with a high ceiling, such as a garage with exposed rafters, securing a metal pole on chains from the beams high enough so your feet cannot touch the floor when fully extended will expand your options. Leg raises are one of the best ab exercises. If you have a weak grip, elbow slings can be purchased inexpensively online that hang from the bar: your weight is supported by your upper arms resting comfortably in the slings, alleviating strain on hands and joints. But eventually you will want to hang by your hands, at least some of the time, as your goal is ultimately about becoming stronger, including hand strength.

Pull-ups are challenging and require strength, so keeping your feet on a stool as an assist is the best way to begin, until you can gauge your strength. Pay heed to any weight limitations of the bar as revealed on the packaging. No matter what the exercise, the same advice applies. It's not the weight, or the type of machine, or the particular exercise that you do; it's how you perform the movement.

When performing biceps curls for example, whether you choose to perform them on a machine, or with cables, a heavy barbell, or light dumbbells, the basic tenants are exactly the same.

If You Want A Flat Tummy, Wear A Belt.

Wearing a weight lifting belt not only supports the back and reminds you to maintain good posture, but it holds in your gut as well. Hard to breathe, you say? That's the point: if your weight training belt makes it hard to breathe, it's because you're breathing incorrectly, through your abdomen, rather than your diaphragm. A weight belt will not affect your breathing if you are breathing correctly by filling your lungs with air, rather than your abdomen.

We're supposed to be inflating our lungs as we breathe, not our bellies, so look down regularly to make sure your belly does not inflate with each breath.

A snug weight lifting belt will be a constant reminder to breathe correctly: you want a small waist, not a big waist.

A snug weight lifting belt will be a constant reminder to pull in and hold in your abdominals, which is not just an exercise in good posture, but a great isometric exercise in itself.

In addition, do not use weights when you train abs. Crunches, leg lifts, hanging leg raises and all other ab exercises should be done without added weights or resistance. Using weights for ab exercises will not increase fat-burning selectively around the waist area, as many erroneously believe.

Keep your waist small by *not* increasing the volume of your abdominal muscles.

The best way to accomplish a small waist is via your diet.

I Know You Won't Listen To Me, Buddy, But That Weight's Too Heavy For You.

When some moron in the gym who is half my size wants to bench press 300 lbs. to feed his ego, and asks me to put myself in jeopardy by spotting him, I say "I don't spot". Sometimes the gym literally falls silent, because spotting stupid people who have no idea what they are doing is supposed to be required gym "etiquette". Not for me it's not.

I will also not spot bodybuilders who are strangers to me but who most likely *do know* what they are doing, either. I will never put myself at risk for an unknown quantity, and that is based on unfortunate experiences, both my own, and those of others around me who have learned the hard way.

I never require or ask anyone for a spot. I only train with the amount of weight that I can handle correctly, because anything more than that is putting me at risk of injury and is counter-productive to building strength and muscle size.

From the opposite perspective of asking someone to spot me, how stupid would I have to be to trust an unknown quantity to do his part if I did lose control of that weight? Do I want the bar crushing my throat because I asked someone who wasn't capable or attentive or experienced enough to rescue me?

And what about people who are spotting their buddies yet are actually doing half the work for them? Whose workout is it, anyway? What's that supposed to accomplish? The idea is for YOU to perform the exercise to YOUR target muscle's fullest ability. Anything less and you are cheating yourself out of optimum results and delaying reaching your goal.

When I do team up with a workout partner, it's with someone compatible who shares my experience and outlook. That means neither of us is attempting to "lift" more than we can handle, because we are not powerlifting. We are bodybuilding. We are performing exercises to build, strengthen and sculpt. We are not trying for a world record, or to impress others. We are not lifting weights: we are *exercising* with weights.

If you can't handle the weight, with your own muscles, all by yourself, that should be a clue that you're headed for danger.

Lifting too heavy a weight means you are cheating yourself out of growth while courting injury at the same time. There's a good reason why you rarely see 60-year-old bodybuilders at the gym. Most guys sustain gym membership-canceling injury before they ever hit 30. And probably 4 out of 5 can blame the bench press for that.

How Much Can You Bench?

This is the question most asked of me when I am in contest

condition. Strangers walk up to me and ask, "How much can you bench press?". I reply, "I don't bench press." They look confused.

How the barbell bench press became the bench mark of weight training I'll never know, as no weightlifting exercise has caused more injury or killed more people.

Forget that it's pretty much a waste of energy due to the fact that 98% of all people use their shoulders to perform what is supposed to be a chest exercise.

The bench press is the alpha male show-off exercise, an ego booster and ego boaster that's supposed to impress everyone watching and prove something extraordinary about the person executing it. However, some end up executing *themselves*, as Sanford Johnson almost did.

USC tailback Johnson was performing the bench press when he lost control of the bar and it landed on his throat. Reportedly he was benching 275 lbs. USC officials stated that an assistant strength and conditioning coach was spotting Johnson when the accident occurred, but was unable to stop the bar from injuring the player.

It goes without saying that if someone you know well who has a vested interest in your staying healthy and vital, and who is also a "strength coach" for a major university football team no less, is unable to rescue you when you get into trouble, what does that say about guys who ask complete strangers to spot them?

A trauma expert who was part of the team that performed over seven hours of throat surgery on him said that Johnson would make a full recovery and be back in the game when healed.

I can't decide on which is the stronger message in this story: don't barbell bench press, or don't spot.

Arms

Why is it that some muscular guys have big blobby arms that have no shape, and others have arms with amazing shape, angles, planes, and cuts, with biceps split down the middle, a high biceps peak, horseshoe triceps and a prominent brachialis anticus?

It's all in their exercise form.

I am always seeing guys at the gym doing biceps curls without fully stretching the biceps at the bottom of the movement, or fully contracting them at the top. They are using too heavy a weight to be able to do these things, as they believe the way to big arms is big weight. They just swing the weight up and down quickly somewhere within a mid-range. This may build size, but they have no definition separating the muscles because their form is so poor, the arc of their movement is truncated, and there is no true mind-to-muscle connection.

People who perform their set really fast are just trying to get it over with…the weight's so heavy, they're afraid they are going to drop it. Or the exercise is so uncomfortable for them, they want it over with ASAP. That attitude is not going to help bring about their goals any faster.

Stretching the biceps fully at the bottom of the arc is uncomfortable, and the movement has to be controlled and slowed down to avoid elbow injury —or worse, a detached biceps requiring surgery and long reovery time— and to maximize results. You cannot hyper extend the arm and elbow at the bottom of the arc, because the biceps will need to disengage from the exercise to accomplish that, and hyper extending can lead to serious injury. Keeping the biceps flexed throughout all ten reps is uncomfortable, both mentally and physically, as lactic acid builds up and causes a burning sensation. But this same uncomfortable burn that is felt deep within the biceps (but certainly should not be felt in the elbow) is what those of us who want to attain growth strive for. This is what "go for the burn" means.

Additionally, flexing, or in other words isometrically squeezing, the biceps forcefully at the top of the movement, and pausing there for a split second to achieve a complete hard flex before seamlessly and fluidly lowering the weight again, is very uncomfortable, and mentally challenging as well. And keeping the biceps flexed throughout all ten reps, well, that requires real concentration and focus. It can be very uncomfortable the first few times you achieve that. But when you witness the physical change it brings, you begin to not only embrace the discomfort, you strive to experience it.

How To Flex: Strike A Pose

You may not realize how intensive and exhausting an on-stage bodybuilder's posing routine is. He is contracting his muscles intensely, flexing with everything he's got, segueing from one muscle group to another, in his attempt to display each muscle group prominently in order to make it stand out and display his hard-won gains.

Some golden advice for you, advice that will ace your workouts and launch you on your way to building and shaping your arms, legs, chest and everything else in record time, is to strike a few poses at home in the privacy of your own mirror.

Posing provides practice in helping you learn how to isolate specific muscles independent of surrounding muscles. This *isolation*, the ability to single out and flex an individual muscle or muscle group, is the KEY to getting the most out of every rep of every exercise you do.

Strike a classic double biceps bodybuilder pose in the bathroom mirror —you know, the one that everybody who is imitating a bodybuilder does, upper arms parallel to the floor, elbows bent, fists pointing to the ceiling... but do it without clenching your fists. Flex your biceps *from the biceps*, not from your hands by squeezing your fists as hard as you can. Practice the double biceps pose open-handed, training your biceps to flex high and proud without squeezing your fists. Your goal is to contract the biceps so strongly that they burn, while keeping the rest of your muscles comparatively relaxed. By doing this, you are learning to isolate the biceps muscle without undue strain or risk of injury.

Next, move your arms into the same position they would be in if performing a biceps curl exercise, and go through the motion of that exercise, without any weight, while trying to duplicate the same burning contraction you achieved while doing the double biceps flexing pose. It's the same pose, the same movement, only done at different angle.

The next time you are getting ready to do biceps curl exercises at home or the gym, first lightly curl your hand around the bar before picking up the weight, FLEX the biceps powerfully, then lift off. Keep the biceps flexed during the entire 10 reps, but pretend you are executing your biceps pose rather than doing a biceps curl exercise. It's all in your mind: you are keeping your focus off moving the weight itself, and onto the sensation of the biceps flexing. You are launching the weight into motion NOT with your hands, but with your biceps, by flexing them. The engine for propelling the weight is not located in your hands; it is located in your biceps.

Remember, flex your biceps immediately before beginning the movement, then, as you perform the curl, remove your attention from the weight, from the bar, and from your hand, and in your mind recreate the feeling of flexing in the mirror open-handed.

Flex, or contract, the biceps to propel the weight when you perform biceps exercises, rather than pulling the weight upward with your hands.

This is mental trickery. Keep the biceps flexed and controlled on the negative portion of the movement, *using the flexed biceps to put the brakes on* as the weight descends, not your hands or shoulders.

Essentially, you are performing a biceps pose with a weight in your hand; disregard the weight and concentrate on achieving the same feeling and sensation in your biceps as you did at home in the mirror. If you perform the exercise too fast, or with too heavy a weight, you will not be able to put the brakes on in a safe and productive way. Stay in control of the weight at all times, or else the weight will control you, and lead you to injury. We are not lifting weights. We are exercising with weights.

Your biceps will grow twice as fast if you just spend a couple of minutes a day flexing, each day trying to hold the flex a little longer, forcing the biceps up a little higher. This in itself is an isometric exercise.

This phenomenon is called the *mind-muscle connection*, whereby just as much effort is going into the mental part of the exercise as the physical. Any pro bodybuilder will tell you that his workouts are at least as mentally draining as they are physically draining.

A mindless workout will yield minor results. Stay focused, and no matter what exercise you are executing, pay close attention to how your flexed target muscle feels throughout the arc of each rep, and throughout each rep of each set. In the beginning, this kind of intense attention and focus can be mentally draining.

Mirror-practice being able to flex and isolate your pecs at home as well, then carry what you've learned into the gym. Get into position to do a chest press, curl your hands lightly round the dumbbells or machine handles, flex your pecs strongly, then immediately lift off. Maintain the flex in your pecs for all ten reps, forcing your pecs to support he weight rather than your shoulders, especially at the top of the exercise, where you'll give the pecs a good squeeze, to remind them that they are the driving force behind propelling the weights.

The number one mistake people make when working their chest is allowing their shoulders to take over and bear the stress that is meant for the pecs. *It's not a shoulder exercise, it's a pec exercise.* Allowing surrounding muscles to help move the weight cheats your primary muscle group out of the results intended for it.

Additionally, at the top of this movement, do not straighten out your arms completely: keep a slight bend in the elbows. Locking your elbows with arms fully extended at the top of this movement will steal the stress from the pecs, where it rightly needs to be in order to build and shape those muscles, and transfers it to your locked shoulder and elbow joints, where it is wasted and potentially injurious. Successfully re-engaging your pectoral muscles from this locked joint position to a full-flex while supporting the dumbbells overhead will be very difficult. You need to keep your pecs flexed/contracted throughout the entire set of repetitions, performed seamlessly and fluidly. As the weights descend, feel your pec muscles themselves resist the heaviness of the weight, not your hands or shoulders. Maintain the stress on your still-flexed pectoral muscles, and stretch your pecs, rather than your shoulders or shoulder joints, in a controlled manner at the bottom of the exercise, before immediately and fluidly powering up into the next rep using only the strength in your pecs to do that.

Learn how to squeeze/flex/contract your pecs by doing so at home in front of the mirror, with no weight in your hand. Soon your progress from performing your chest exercises correctly will become infinitely more evident.

Even as you sit at the computer you can flex your back, calves, thighs, etc. Get familiar with all your muscles and learn how to isolate them safely at home without weights so your time at the gym will yield faster and more impressive results. As you read this, you can practice flexing the muscles we are talking about. You should be able to flex/contract any given muscle in your body from whatever physical position you may be in right now: sitting at your desk, lying on your bed, standing in front of a mirror, or curled up on the couch.

The more you practice flexing, the better at isolating the target muscles when doing your workout exercises you will become, and the greater and faster your progress. I love the gym, but I don't want to be there any longer than I have to be.

Watch most guys when they are doing a barbell bench press at the gym, especially if they go heavy: they are using their shoulders to bear the brunt of the weight, rather than their pecs. When you learn to flex and isolate your pecs in the mirror, you will perform the barbell bench press and all chest exercises in a whole new productive way, harnessing the flex in your pecs to power the weight up into the positive/ascending movement, and using the flex in your pecs to put the brakes on while performing the negative/descending portion of the movement. Note that because you are now using the correct muscle to perform the chest press exercises, and removing your shoulders from the equation, that you will need to really lighten up on the weight. Your pecs need time to catch up in size and strength with your shoulders. If you perform the bench press correctly in the way described here, you will not be able to handle anywhere near your previous shoulder-driven chest press poundage.

Practice flexing, then lighten that weight up —as you should always do whenever changing things around or trying new things. See what a difference flexing makes in the sensation you have in your pecs after completing your set.

Read Instructions Before Assembling.

Many people seem to believe that the advice of a champion bodybuilder would hold little value for them because their goal is to get fit, not become a bodybuilder. That's like saying Donald Trump's financial advice would hold no value for them because they don't want to become a millionaire, just be financially better-off.

You may not want to look like a champion bodybuilder, but they know the answer to just about any question you might have. They were at one time skinny or fat, and had no idea where to begin or how to achieve their goal. They have solved almost any problem that you yourself will encounter, have injured themselves and rehabbed and recovered, know how to tweak their nutrition to get a certain effect, and have excelled beyond most other peoples' wildest dreams.

When you open a bodybuilding magazine, you may not exactly

like the way he looks, but you'll find a lot to like in what he has to say.

Yes, there are a few knuckleheads in the mix, but most accomplished men and women in the bodybuilding and fitness industry have a wealth of knowledge to share. So take a few minutes to page thru a bodybuilding/fitness magazine or two when you're at the supermarket or newsstand.

If you are female and turned off by the female bodybuilders who are bigger and butcher than most guys are, keep in mind they are a freakish minority. Competitions like the Fitness America Pageant showcase beautiful women in amazing shape who are at the top of the fitness pyramid. Check them out using search engines, or on youtube.com.

Most people who are enthusiastic hobbyists with an interest in carpentry, fly-fishing, doll collecting, etc., are constantly learning. They subscribe to specialty magazines, join online communities, contribute to online forums, attend trade shows, and so on. Their goal is to get better at what they do, meet and socialize with like-minded individuals, and to exchange ideas and tricks of the trade, purchase equipment, and just simply surround themselves with what gives them satisfaction and happiness.

Ironically, most people who go to the gym do none of these things. They don't study magazines or journals, watch instructional video, or attend trade shows. For most, the gym is just another chore to get past so they can check it off their list, which is why they do not succeed or excel.

"I already go to the gym three times a week, that's enough!"

If you expect to change your physique, your state of health and your level of strength, you need to take a focused interest, rather than an casual attitude. You can either go through the motions of knocking together a cabinet in your cellar, or you can research everything you can about cabinet construction, do things right, take a class, seek out the advice of others who are more experienced, and thus construct an heirloom you can be proud of and that will hold you in good stead for decades to come.

It makes no sense that so many people who go to gyms never seek out any instruction: there are instructions posted on the machines, instructions in bodybuilding and fitness magazines, instruction on the DVDs that are playing on gym monitors, instructional DVDs available for rent or purchase, and videos posted free online just by clicking, such as those on <www.bodybuilding.com/fit>

I have belonged to some gyms for years on end that had members I would see continually, year after year, who made no progress whatsoever. I'd love to know how someone gets the motivation to keep going to the gym, and paying his or her fees, when there is no visible change. On the other hand, I have seen people with no development at all join a gym and within six months have entered a fitness or bodybuilding contest. This is not a random phenomenon. The people who make no progress do not know what they are doing, don't seek a solution for that, and don't have any clearly visualized goal in mind.

Another odd phenomenon occurs when someone with impressive development is correctly performing an exercise —let's say dumbbell curls, in the mirror. Next to him stands someone with no development at all, doing the same exercise at the same time, but totally incorrectly. That person seems completely oblivious to the impressively developed guy next to him doing the same exercise, correctly, whose form he might try to imitate. It makes me think about one of the catch-phrases of the '60s: *Be Here Now*. Many people at the gym are simply not present. They're off in the clouds, just going through the motions.

To spend the time and effort to work out, for months or years on end, and pay money for a gym membership, and never make the effort to learn anything about the process, is crazy.

The Weight Itself Is Secondary

It is extremely important to understand that the amount of weight and the weight object itself are secondary to the proper performance of the exercise. This means that the weight is simply an object of resistance, a tool to challenge the target muscle, a means to an end, and nothing more.

We are not powerlifting, we are strength training. We are not trying to lift the heaviest weight we possibly can; we are exercising, building and sculpting our muscles using the weights as our tool.

Keep your focus off the weight, and on the target muscle.

Where Is My Target Muscle?

Your target muscle is the muscle or muscle group that any particular exercise is designed to challenge.

It is vital to know why you are doing each particular exercise and which muscle or muscle group each exercise is intended to target.

In most gyms, exercise machines have an anatomical illustration that highlights in red the muscles that the machine targets. But you need to go beyond this and read or watch videos so that you will gain more extensive knowledge. Often people approach me at the gym and ask exactly what the exercise I am performing is for. Often an exercise they thought I was doing for shoulders was actually for the back, for example, even though there is a diagram on the machine itself that tells them the machine is designed for a back exercise. I have also observed people asking this question of others, and receiving an incorrect answer, because the person performing the exercise did not know himself what muscle the exercise was intended to target.

Knowing the target muscle for every exercise is crucial so that the exercise can be performed correctly, so that exercises will not be duplicated, wasting your time, so that the proper muscles can be flexed at the outset of the exercise, and most importantly, so you will see impressive progress as quickly as possible.

Keeping the target muscle flexed, or engaged, during the entire movement will shift your progress into overdrive. We can work out in a lazy inattentive manner, or we can stay focused and intensely involved. Both take the exact same amount of time, but staying focused gives us far faster, superior results.

Your Hands Are Merely Handles

Most people lag, or even fail at strength training because they place all their focus and attention on the weight instead of on the target muscle.

It is the contraction, or flexing, of the target muscle, rather than your hands, that propels the weight into motion.

In everyday life we rarely isolate our pecs or our calves, for example, to perform any particular task. The body instead calls up every available muscle to form a team to perform any given job, such as putting a heavy box on a high shelf. The shoulders, abs, pecs, back, calves, quads…and much more…all work in tandem to accomplish this one particular task.

But in strength training, it's the exact opposite. The muscles are no longer team players. We intentionally perform tasks, or exercises, that isolate each muscle or muscle group individually to stress it in a concentrated way, unlike anything we normally would do in day-to-day situations.

It is this isolation that makes the muscle quickly strengthen, shape and grow. It is the target muscle that must drive each individual exercise, not the hands holding the weights. Your hands are simply handles, devices that connect the weight to your body so your target muscle can work against the weight's resistant force.

It's important that as long as you're making the time and effort to do it, that you commit to doing it right. Often I see people at the gym who have paid their money, gotten dressed, set aside the time, driven to the gym and then sit on the equipment daydreaming, or halfheartedly go through the motions with no conscious connection to what they are doing. They've already done 95% of what they need to do to get the results they want, then they fail at the one and only thing that really matters: doing the exercise correctly in a focused and deliberate manner with an emotional connection.

Don't watch TV, read, or answer the cell phone while working out. Rest as little as possible between sets and exercises. Time yourself so that, ideally, no more than 2 minutes go by without activity. Listen to your body. If the weight is too heavy, go lighter or do fewer repetitions. If in the beginning you need more than 2 minutes' rest, take it, but keep that 2-minute rest goal in mind for the nearest possible future. Making your strength training aerobic by keeping your heart rate up throughout your workout will increase its overall value, strengthening your heart and lungs along with your arms and abs, and burning fat as well... a true win/win situation.

The Negative Is A Very Positive Thing

In every strength training exercise, the **ascent,** or the raising of the weight from the starting position, is called the **positive**.

In every strength training exercise, the **descent,** or the lowering of the weight from the apex position, is called the **negative**.

The ascent is the positive. The descent is the negative.

The negative is as crucial and beneficial a part of every exercise as is the positive.

All too often I see people struggle to raise a too-heavy weight, and then allow that weight then to free-fall back to starting position. This free-fall not only puts them in danger of injury, but also cancels out fully half of the exercise's benefits.

Lowering the weight under control against the resistance of the target muscle is just as essential to building strength and muscle and reaching your goals as the raising of the weight is. We are not powerlifting; powerlifting requires only that the participant lifts the weight. After accomplishing that, he literally throws the weight out of the way. A powerlifter wouldn't dream of lowering the weight safely or in a controlled manner to the floor, because it's too damn heavy. Most males who work out at gyms confuse powerlifting with bodybuilding: the two disciplines are apples and oranges.

Never throw away the negative. If you're *that* tired or your muscles are *that* spent, then switch to a lighter weight that you will be in full control of, or do fewer reps. Nobody wants to hear your weights slam to the gym floor, especially the owner.

Slowly count one-two-three as you perform the positive portion of every exercise, squeeze and contract the target muscle for a split second at the top of the exercise, and then slowly count one-two-three-four on the descent or negative portion of the exercise. If you can perform the negative portion of the exercise even slower than the positive portion, you'll be carving even more shape into the muscle.

Remember, it's the shape and contours of the muscle that makes your arms, legs and other parts look big, impressive, pretty, or powerful …not just their actual measured size. When I was at my heaviest muscle weight in my early 50s, almost 200 pounds, I was watching a bodybuilding contest on TV. One of my favorite bodybuilders, Tito Raymond, came on stage looking phenomenal, big, but very symmetrical, tight and cut. "Much better than me", I thought.

Then they flashed his stats on the screen: we were the same height, yet how could someone who looked so awesome, who looked bigger than I, weigh just 176 lbs. —almost 25 pounds less than me? How did he manage to look bigger than I did? Again it was a valuable lesson for me, as I began to see this become a pattern in contests when I began paying closer attention to the personal stats, these awesome-looking physiques that made the contestant look far bigger than his weight indicated. Two days after this, I saw Tito at Gold's gym in Venice, and in a sweatshirt he didn't look anything like he had on stage, but soon he took the shirt off to reveal the same structure I had seen when he was in that contest.

It was the illusion created by symmetry, proportion and muscle definition. He concentrated on building certain muscles larger while keeping others, especially his core muscles, small, defined and tight. He looked powerfully built onstage, yet his overall body size in fact was compact.

Females not interested in size are surely interested in shape, so women should work out accordingly, deliberately executing each movement. This is what carves shape. The poundage you are using, light or heavy, will determine muscle size.

Utilizing light weights, along with perfect form and focused mind-to-muscle connection, will create beautifully shaped petite muscle in females and compact muscle in males.

Using heavy weights along with perfect form with focused mind-to-muscle connection (and increasing your intake of good muscle-building food) will create beautifully shaped big muscle.

If you go heavy, keep in mind that if you are not in control of the weight, the weight will be in control of you. And that spells injury.

Core Strength

Your abdominal and lower back muscles provide core stability, balance and strength. No exercises are more important to lifelong pain-free overall mobility than abs and lower back exercises. Every movement you make, from picking up a child to washing the car —not to mention working out— depends on core strength. If you do nothing else on a "feelin' lazy" day, at least work abs and lower back for core strength and stability.

Since you're not trying to build size in these areas, you can work them any or every day. But when they do get sore, take off a day or two to rest until the soreness has subsided.

Muscles tone, change shape and grow *while we are at rest*, not while we are working out.

Give them the time off they need for fastest progress.

Overtraining is not some myth, it's a fact. If you become obsessed with working out and don't take enough rest days, your body never gets the chance to fully rebuild the muscle properly, to make full use of all that work you just did during your workout. We tear down the muscle fibers at the gym. They rebuild while we are at rest, and while we sleep.

Chapter 5
**Your Strength Training Workout Routine:
Exercises and Advice**

Contained in this section is a lot of crucial information concerning re-thinking your form and flow, some of which may initially go over the heads of beginners, but will resonate with those who have spent many hours in their home gym or health club.

If you cannot invest time or money in a gym membership and have limited resources for equipment, there's actually quite a bit you can do at home. Following is a list of mostly mainstream, well-known strength training exercises that you can perform with minimal equipment. The more time you spend on the Internet browsing workout and exercise videos, the more options you will find for each muscle group. For example, you may not like a particular shoulder exercise, but may enjoy performing a different variation of it.

Remember, exercises done without resistance, either the resistance that your own body weight provides, or resistance provided by weights, will yield minimal results. To see impressive gains faster, choose resistance exercises over aerobics or cardio. Perform them slowly & deliberately, using an amount of weight you can readily handle, to attain a rewarding result and enjoy freedom from injury.

Browse The Internet

Enter the exercise terms that you see set in boldface type in this section into a search engine to find dozens of videos for each exercise. There are many, many sources online, among them mayoclinic.com, youtube.com, bodybuilding.com, and about.com. Some present better examples than others, but the more you search the more you'll discover good quality videos that provide clear visuals, explained in plain language, although the truly outstanding are few and far between. With over 50 possible exercises for each muscle group, it would take a monumental effort to produce quality instruction for each and every one.

My own **WORKOUT PhD** DVD presents a selection of strength training exercises with very detailed instructions for how to perform them and what you should be feeling as you perform them. The principals explained in my DVD are meant to be applied to every strength training exercise there is: the principles of flexing and extending the target muscle without involving surrounding muscles or impacting joints, are designed to be applied to all exercises. You can view free clips and order my DVD here:

http://www.discoveringhawaii.com

Click on *Fitness* in the menu at the top of the page.

Choice Is Everything

You may find a particular biceps curl exercise difficult,

uncomfortable and frustrating, yet find another version enjoyable, satisfying and productive. Browsing around on youtube.com, bodybuilding.com and various exercise sites will unlock for you, as they have for me, a whole world of exercises and fresh tips on performing them. Our education never ceases.

Change Is Good

I change my routine almost every workout, based on tedium, or energy level, or a perceived slowdown in progress; whether I'm feeling any pain or rigidity in the muscle or surrounding joints, or to surprise and jolt my muscles into new growth. Our bodies can become accustomed to the same old same old. Our muscles and bones need fresh challenges in order to regenerate and grow optimally stronger, faster.

It is crucial to understand that the *engine* that drives your exercise is housed within the target muscle and not in your hand, not in the weight, and not in any surrounding muscle groups.

It isn't the wheels that propel your car, it's the engine housed under the hood. The wheels are merely objects that connect the vehicle with the road. The wheels don't propel the car; the engine does.

Your focus on feeling what is transpiring within the target muscle as you perform the movement must be as strong as your focus on correct form and execution. It may look like you are performing the exercise the correct way, but only if you are driving the exercise from the target muscle itself will you feel it the way you should, from deep within the target muscle, and thus derive the utmost benefit in the least amount of time.

For your home workout routine, you'll need 3 items: a pair of dumbbells, a flat bench such as a commercial weight bench, picnic bench or ottoman, and a door frame chin-up bar. You may find this equipment at a discount store like Wal-Mart or Costco, at a garage sale, in The Pennysaver or Recycler newspapers or on their websites, or on craigslist.com.

Your Workout Routine

The word REP means repetition. A SET is made up of a number of REPS, ideally between 8 and 12 reps. We need to do between 3 and 4 sets of each exercise.

For example, if you choose Push-ups from the menu below, you need to complete between 8 and 12 REPS of this exercise to comprise a good SET, and complete a total of 3 or 4 SETS before you move on to the next exercise.

If you choose Triceps Extensions from the menu below, you need to complete between 8 and 12 REPS of this exercise to comprise a good SET, and complete a total of 3 or 4 SETS before you move on to the next exercise.

Less is okay for beginners, but these numbers should be your eventual goal.

In a few months, when our abilities become polished and we hit our stride, we can rearrange our workout so that we work each major group —arms, chest, legs, etc.— just once a week, but intensely so.

"Intense" means that you will be able to fully complete 9-12 strong, focused, challenging SETS for each body part. That means 9-12 sets for arms, 9-12 sets for chest, etc.

Doing the math, this means you will be performing 3 SETS of 3 different biceps exercises, for a total of 9 SETS for the biceps.

This means when exercising your pecs, you will perform 3 sets each of 3 different pec exercises, for a total of 9 Sets.

When a muscle group is taxed to its capacity, it will need a full week's rest —or more— *and* optimum nutrition to fully recover and transform. Our muscles grow, shape, and strengthen during this rest period, *not* while we are in the gym.

Muscle and bone require quality food to grow, re-shape and strengthen. The workout itself effectively tears down muscle tissue so that it can rebuild even stronger and firmer while we rest, and eat. So after intense workouts, our bodies need a full week to do this job of rebuilding. This is why, as you become more advanced, you will graduate to working just one body part per session, —your arms for example, so that your arms will have a full week to repair and rebuild before you work arms gain.

By scheduling just one body part per workout session, it will allow you to completely focus on that body part only, producing optimum results. You will also allow that body part a full week to rest, repair itself, and rejuvenate.

When I was 48 years old, I read an article in one of the bodybuilding magazines by Bill Davey, who fully explained his own (new to me) one-body-part-a-day routine, and illustrated it with inspirational photographs of what he had accomplished. I had not made satisfactory gains in some time, after enjoying periods of growth, and I personally need to see progress in order to stay enthused. So I gave the one-bodypart-per-session routine a try. I was astonished at the jump start it gave my physique. It truly opened the door to greater results, and I have stayed with this program to this day. A five-session schedule would include working chest on day 1, arms on day 2, legs on day 3, shoulders on day 4, and back on day 5, not necessarily in that order.

My own schedule is a six-session schedule:

Day 1: Chest
Day 2: Arms
Day 3: Hamstrings, Calves and Glutes
Day 4: Back
Day 5: Shoulders
Day 6: Quadriceps (Thighs) and Calves.

I split my leg workout into two sessions, and spread those leg days as far apart as I can, because an intense leg workout is exhausting, and requires a lot of energy and recovery time. If I do an entire leg workout in just one session, I have to cut down on both the number of sets, and exercises.

I do repeat working my calves on the second leg day, but I do different calf exercises each time. My calves respond well to this, after years of disappointing growth, which was due mostly to lack of effort on my part. Originally I decided to work calves twice a week because I actually hated working calves, and I thought this would make it easier on me. You know, less effort, less drudge, such was my thinking. But when I finally saw them growing, they became my new favorite body part to work, and working them intensely two sessions out of six gave me great results. I may take as long as 11 days to complete a six-session workout. A six-session workout does not mean working out six days in a row. You need rest. I have worked out six days in a row a few times, when greatly enthused, or when in need of the stress relief that workouts bring, but rarely do I ever complete a 6-session work out within a 7 or 8 day period.

I listen to my body, and when it says it needs rest, I rest. I know from experience that I make great progress with intense workouts and lots of rest days in between. When I am in a committed period, such as when I am trying to get into contest shape, I try not to take a holiday from working out that lasts more than 3 days, however.

I do not have a typical routine. I never repeat the exact workout twice. The gym has a lot of different machines, and I try to make use of them all. But in the following chapters concerning what I eat and what I do at the gym, I will outline many of the exercises that I do most often.

Beginners and those who have not worked out in a long time can choose one exercise from each group (Chest, Triceps, Back, etc.) in the Exercise Menu list that follows.

Absolute Beginners who are unsure about all this, can skip down to the **Are You An Absolute Beginner?** section for a ten-exercise routine.

Again, entering the terms below seen in bold type into a search engine will reveal dozens of short videos that will show better than almost any still image could, how to proceed.

Remember, you need to work out three days a week no matter what your primary goal is, whether it be to attain the aerobic and cardio benefits, or to attain the strength and beauty benefits. As you become stronger, you can add more exercises for each muscle group, for a total of 3 or 4 exercises for each group. Eventually, when you are seeing continued impressive results, you can switch to a single-body part-per-day schedule with rest days factored in as needed.

Those who have trouble viewing videos on their computer because the video is jumpy, or starts and stops continually, can greatly benefit from purchasing additional memory for their computer. Additional memory has never been more powerful, or cheaper. Sometimes these problems have to do with your internet access provider, and how fast a connection they are able to provide. Shop around for the fastest provider.

Exercise Menu

Chest

—**Push-ups** performed between two chairs; place one hand on each chair seat, with hands spaced wide. This works outer pecs. Hands spaced close together works inner pecs.
—Push-ups from the floor with hands spaced close together. This works inner pecs. Hands placed farther apart works outer pecs.
—Push-ups from a higher raised surface, such as the back of a sofa, or a railing. This is good for those who are just beginning, or who experience discomfort when doing boot-camp style push-ups.
—**Flat bench dumbbell presses** lying on a bench, ottoman or the floor. Primarily builds size.
—**Flat bench dumbbell flyes** lying on a bench, ottoman, or the floor. Primarily builds shape.
—**Dumbbell Pullover** builds size and shape by working/stretching the pecs in a vertical axis, while the other exercises above work on a horizontal axis.

Remarks: Isolate your pecs by practicing flexing them in a mirror. Isolating body parts does not come naturally to most people, and trying to do so for the first time with heavy weights in your hands is not a good idea. Flex your pecs forcefully immediately before beginning the movement, and maintain the flex throughout. This takes real concentration and practice, but the payoff in terms of results will be greater.

Dumbbell pullovers should be done in a very controlled manner. When you bring the weight behind your head, flex your pecs and stretch only the pecs. It is easy to hyper-extend and involve the shoulder joints, allowing the dumbbell to extend behind your head even further, but this will be of no benefit to your pec development and may injure your shoulders. At the top of the exercise, the dumbbell should be hovering directly over your pecs. Concentrate at this point to make sure all the stress is on your pecs, by flexing them emphatically and maintaining that flex as you move fluidly and seamlessly into the next rep.

Back

—**Chin-up/pull-up** bar: chin-up / Pull up with palms facing toward you.
—**Chin-up/pull-up** bar: chin-up / Pull up with palms facing away from you.
—**Wide-grip chin-up** with palms facing away from you to target latissimus muscles.
—**Assisted chin-ups**: all the above performed while you place one or both feet on a stable stool or chair, so that your full weight does not stress your shoulder joints.
—**Dumbbell bent row**
—**Dumbbell bent over reverse flyes**
—**Dumbbell dead lift**

Remarks: Get into position, wrap your hands around the handles, then flex your back emphatically and in a focused manner before picking up the dumbbells and beginning any back movement. Keep your back flexed and your core stabilized during the entire set of repetitions.

Pull-ups: Do not allow your arms to fully extend as you hang: keep your lats and back muscles flexed and always keep a slight bend in your elbows. Hyper-extending your arms deletes your back muscles from the entire equation, putting most of the stress on your joints, and when attempting to re-engage the muscles, injury becomes a greater possibility. Keep the reps fluid and seamless. Do not jerk yourself up when you begin to tire: simply stop at that point. The whole idea is to challenge your back muscles to do all the work. Any cheat, like lurching or jerking movements, will rob your back of its potential growth and open the door to injury. It's not how many reps you do; it's the quality of your execution. If you can only do two focused reps, then good for you: in a week or two you'll be able to do three. Then four. Injure yourself, and you won't be able to do *any*.

Dumbbell deadlifts are an outstanding lower back and core exercise, but if done incorrectly can lead to lower back injury. Watch as many different videos as you can locate in order to get the best examples of how this exercise should be performed. Attempt it the first time with no weights in your hands. Stabilize your core and do not allow your spine to curve. Flex your butt powerfully as you return to an upright position, and keep the butt flexed on the negative as well. Doing so will help keep your core stable and tight.

Triceps

—**Triceps kick-backs**, single dumbbell
—**One-arm Triceps extensions**, seated with single dumbbell
—One-armed Triceps extensions, lying with on your back on a bench or floor, with single dumbbell
—**Triceps bench-dips**

Remarks: You may find that learning to keep constant tension in your triceps is even more of a challenge than keeping constant tension in your biceps, because we've had less practice doing that.

—First grasp the dumbbell.
— Second, flex the triceps.

—Third, begin the movement.

Keep your triceps flexed during the entire set of fluid, seamless repetitions. Avoid jerky movements. There should be no pause between reps in any of the exercises you do.

Power the dumbbell upward by engaging the engine that is housed within your triceps, not by merely forcing your hand into motion: keep your focus on the target muscle itself, not on the dumbbell, or on your hand.

Your hands are merely handles that attach you to the weight: this is their only function.

Keep your triceps muscles flexed, stretching them as you descend on the negative, then flexing powerfully on the positive in order to power the weight upward. Avoid stretching too far at the bottom, or a painful elbow problem may present itself: this is not an elbow exercise, it is a triceps exercise.

Keep your elbow joints out of the equation. If you are feeling any strain or pain in the elbow, you may be stretching too far on the negative, but for sure your triceps are not bearing the full stress of the exercise: you are allowing your elbow joint to become involved. Think only of and about your triceps muscles while performing triceps exercises.

At the top of the movement, never lock your elbows. Locking the elbows puts undue strain on them and steals the energy away from the triceps needed to grow and change their shape: the whole point of any exercise is to keep constant stress/tension *on the muscle* you are trying to build, and *off your joints*.

Many people lock their elbows at the top of the movement in

order to take a split-second's rest before beginning the next rep. Don't do that. There is no resting. If you can only do 4 or 5 perfect reps, that's far better than doing 10 bad reps. As you grow stronger, you will be able to increase the number of perfectly executed reps.

There should be no beginning or end to a rep. Instead there should be a smooth, fluid seamless transition from one rep to another, as if your arm is attached to a large rubber band. Six fluid, seamless, elegant reps will provide greater and safer results than will 8 or 10 jerky, joint-stressing reps.

Triceps bench-dips: Get into position, and then flex your triceps emphatically, with elbows bent, before lowering your body. Do not hyper-extend at the bottom of the movement, and do not lock your elbows or shoulder joints at the top: always keep a slight bend in the elbow. This will place more stress exactly where you want it...*on the triceps*, and less where you don't...on the joints.

Biceps

—Biceps **alternating dumbbell curls**, standing
—Biceps **alternating dumbbell curls**, seated
—**One Arm Prone Dumbbell Curl**: can be done standing, bent forward at waist with weighted arm hanging freely and the other supporting your body, or on an incline bench.
—**One Arm Prone Dumbbell Curl**: dumbbell curls performed over an ottoman (lie on your stomach on the ottoman with the edge hitting you in your armpit, arm extending over airspace, allowing biceps to lower dumbbell toward the floor). If using a bench, cushion your triceps with a rolled up towel.

Remarks: Pose in the mirror before beginning your biceps routine so you can familiarize yourself with the feel of a good hard flex in your biceps without the distraction of having a dumbbell in your hand. Keep that sensation in your mind when you do take a dumbbell in your hand so you will stay on track and not involve your hands or shoulders in this exercise.

Biceps exercises are for biceps only, and biceps are a tiny enough muscle group as it is...so any cheating the weight up you may be tempted to do just robs the biceps out of the growth they'd normally enjoy if the exercise were performed strictly. Use an amount of weight you can readily handle.

—First, grasp the dumbbell.
—Second, flex your biceps.
—Third, power up by flexing the biceps and perform the exercise, keeping constant tension on the biceps throughout the entire set of reps.

On the negative, never hyper-extend the arm or elbow. Keep a slight bend in the elbow. With the biceps flexed on the negative portion, stretch the biceps as far as you are comfortable with, *without involving the elbow joint.*

Men who have built big arms lacking in definition typically do not perform biceps curls with a full range of motion. They do not flex emphatically at the top of the movement, nor stretch the biceps fully (the biceps, not the elbow) at the bottom of the movement. They limit themselves to a truncated range of motion somewhere in the middle, with heavy weights. Not performing the exercise with a full range of motion with a weight you can readily handle will rob you of the classic shape associated with great arms.

If doing these or any exercises properly and in a controlled manner is "too difficult" it's because the weight is "too heavy".

Lighten up and do it right. Once your biceps become accustomed to handling all the stress associated with this movement, they will strengthen, and you will then be able to add more weight.

It's only human: we hate having to interrupt our flow by correcting our form and basically re-training ourselves to do a familiar exercise. But any perceived loss of progress will be quickly made up for and then surpassed with new, faster development once we learn to maximize each exercise.

Forearms

—**Reverse curls**
—**Hammer curls**
—**Wrist curls**, palms up
—**Wrist curls**, palms down

Remarks: *The wrist curl is not a wrist exercise,* despite the inaccurate common name given it.

Over-stretching or hyper-extending your wrist on the negative will just give you a painful wrist. This is a forearm exercise, and flexing the forearm at the top of the movement, powerfully, and getting a good, slow, controlled eccentric, or negative, will pump up your forearms fast. The reason most people don't see results after doing a forearm routine is because they are over-extending their wrists and under-flexing their forearms. On the negative portion of the exercise, concentrate on, and stretch the forearm muscles in a slow and controlled manner, and when you get to the point in the negative where you feel more wrist strain than forearm strain, you've extended too far.

Hammer curls performed one arm at a time, with the dumbbell arching over your pec on the positive, rather than raising straight up and down at a 180 degree angle, will include involvement of your brachialis, giving you more bang for your buck. If you'd rather exercise both arms at once (you won't be able to cross over this way, though), sit on a bench or stool if standing causes you to rock too much.

Reverse curls can be performed by kneeling on a folded towel in front of the bench/ottoman, laying your arms palm down on the bench/ottoman while grasping the dumbbell, flexing the forearm hard, and raising the weight, but not the elbow. Keep your elbow touching the bench. The engine for raising the dumbbell is housed in your forearm, not your shoulder, or hand, or wrist. Forget about your hand, forget about the dumbbell: keep your mind on the forearm and how it feels, especially near the top of the movement. Find the sweet spot where it doesn't hurt, stop there for a split second, flex hard, them fluidly and immediately slowly lower the weight to just barely touching the ottoman/bench, then immediately, seamlessly, deliberately and fluidly raise it up again.

Abs

—**Hanging Leg raises** from the chin-up bar, knees bent to clear floor.
—**Abdominal Crunches**
—Flat Bench **Abdominal Leg Pull Ins**
— **Abdominal Side bends**

Remarks: If you have any back problems, avoid all twisting or torquing at the waist.

Many people make the mistake of thinking the goal with crunches is to raise your head and shoulders as high off the floor or bench as possible: they put their hands behind their head and actually yank it upward. Ouch!

The engine powering your abdominal exercises is always, and only, located deep within your abs. Pulling your head up with your hands is not good for your abs, or your neck.

Keep your lower back flat against the floor, then flex your ab muscles, pulling them inward, not pushing them outward. Then curl your torso up using only the flex of your ab muscles, slowly. You are not trying to raise your head and shoulders high off the floor: that is not the point. The point is how hard you can flex your abs, and the challenge of maintaining that flex at the apex, and throughout the entire set.

Keep your ab muscles flexed/pulled in hard throughout all the reps, both on the positive and the negative. This at first may be very challenging for you, and it does take focus and concentration, but we are working to create a flat six-pack, not a convex six-pack.

Even if you only get a crunching movement of a just few degrees off the floor at first, it's a correct start, as doing it wrong will get you nowhere and probably hurt your neck and upper back. Your ab muscles will quickly become stronger, and your ability to flex and hold the flex, more assured and more powerful.

Begin with your back flat on the floor and knees bent or propped on a bench. Flex your lower abs and lower back muscles simultaneously, then curl your torso upward, slowly, deliberately, all the while pulling your abs in, and tensing them hard at the top, then lowering back to starting position, keeping the abs flexed all the while. Even if this is not a new exercise for you, relearning how to do it right will take concentration. Remember: we are not trying to see how high we can curl our torso up…that isn't the point at all. We are challenging ourselves as to how hard and prolonged we can keep our abs flexed as we curl only as far as is comfortable for us.

Side bends, or any ab exercise for that matter, should not be done with a dumbbell or any added weight at all. We do not want to build muscle in our waist; we just want to make the natural muscle we already have there harder, sexier, and more defined. We want a *smaller* waist, not a bigger waist. We want definition, cuts, and firmness in our waist musculature, *not added size*. Using weights will add size where we do not want it.

While I'm thinking of it, posture is everything, and pulling in your abs every time you think of it is not only good posture, but is also a powerful isometric exercise that you can do anywhere, even while driving. Pull in your lower abs, flex them as hard as you can, and do a slow count to six.

Legs

—**Sissy squats**
—**One-legged sissy squats** holding a dumbbell
—**Dumbbell Lunges** (don't allow your knee to extend forward of your toes)
—**Step-ups with dumbbells**
—**Dumbbell Calf Raises** standing on a stair
—**Dumbbell Seated Calf Raises** with dumbbell resting on the knee for resistance.
—**Dumbbell Hamstring Curls**: it is vital to build hamstring strength along with thigh strength, or you'll look weird, and fall over.
—Standing or Lying **Hamstring Curls with ankle weights**.

Remarks: Remember, the engine that drives every exercise we perform is located within the muscle group we are targeting, not in our feet or ankles.

Sissy Squats: Hold onto a chair back or other stable object for balance. Slowly descend, keeping your thighs/quads flexed and putting the breaks on with your butt muscles, not your knees as you get closer to the floor. *Don't descend too deeply*, or too quickly, as this will stress the knees and deprive your quads of the benefit of the exercise. Don't rest at the bottom. Pretend your joints are connected by giant rubber bands, like those old-fashioned jointed dolls, and strive for a smooth, fluid movement, from one rep to another, without pausing.

Power yourself back up smoothly by powerfully flexing your butt muscles. Try not to pause at the top, and don't lock your knees; keep your knees a little bent at the top of the movement, as this will stress your quads nicely and protect your knees from wear and tear. Then, descend again immediately, in a very controlled, fluid, and deliberate manner, keeping the brakes on in your butt and front thigh muscles. Maintain the rubber band analogy to keep stress off your knees. If you can only do 4 perfect reps, then go ahead and do 4 …that's better than doing six or eight poor reps. Strive for 10 quality reps eventually, and when you accomplish that, up the ante to fifteen.

Calf Raises: When you do calf raises, keep your ankles out of the movement. *This is not an ankle exercise.* You stretch and flex only your calves, and never hyper-extend your ankles. That means, you don't challenge yourself to see how far down or how far up on your toes you can stretch, because it will lead to injury and does not enhance muscle growth at all. Do 3 sets of ten repetitions with your feet placed shoulder width apart, and toes pointing inward. Then do

3 sets of ten with your feet shoulder width apart, and toes pointing outward. This variation will add shape to your calves.

Lunges: Never allow your knee to extend further out than, or beyond, your foot when performing the lunge. Doing so will put tremendous stress on the knee, and won't enhance muscle growth one bit. Keep your butt flexed and use your butt as a shock absorber, not your knees.

Lying Hamstring dumbbell curls: Performed on a bench/ottoman. Picking up the dumbbell with your feet takes practice. So perform this the first time with no dumbbell at all so you can get the movement down correctly before proceeding with a weight. Then, perform it again practicing picking up a light object with your feet, such as a 2 lb. dumbbell, or a kid's or dog's toy, just to get the movement down.

Lay the dumbbell on the floor in front of and in line with the bench and straddle the dumbbell with your feet, far enough away from the bench or ottoman so that when you bend your knees and fall forward, in a controlled manner, of course, your knees will be fully supported by the bench, to prevent knee strain or injury. With practice, you can harness the momentum of gently falling forward in order to raise the dumbbell at the same time, saving your knees from the added stress that lifting the weight from a prone body position might cause.

Grab the bench with each hand, flex your butt powerfully, them curl your legs, pulling the dumbbell toward your butt, and then flex your butt and hamstrings hard. Maintain that flex as you slowly lower the dumbbell, but not too far…you want the eccentric / negative stretch to stress your hamstrings, not your knee joints! Go slowly, perform the movement deliberately, and practice it a few times without using a dumbbell just to get it right. This exercise will provide added benefit to your calves as well.

Shoulders

—**Dumbbell Shoulder Raise** to the front, or anterior, one or both arms at a time
   —**Dumbbell Lateral Raise** / to the side
   —**Dumbbell Shoulder Press** overhead
   —**Dumbbell Bent Over Flyes** for rear delts
   —**Dumbbell Upright Row**

Remarks: **Dumbbell Shoulder Press.** First grasp the dumbbell, then flex your shoulders and keep them flexed throughout the exercise. Do not hyper-extend your arms when doing an overhead press: maintain a slight bend in the elbows at the top of the movement. Many trainers want you to maintain a certain hand position or angle, but remember, this is a shoulder exercise and all the power should be driven directly from the shoulder, smoothly and fluidly, not the hands. Allow your hands and dumbbells to rotate into any angle that is comfortable and natural for you.

Are You An Absolute Beginner?

If you have never worked out before, and want to sample a full-body, first-try-it-at-home routine, try this ten-exercise program using a set of 2 lb./0.5k, or 5 lb./2k dumbbells.

Remember, slow and deliberate fluidity will give great results and keep you safe from injury.

Your goal should be three sets of ten repetitions for each exercise.

You can divide this list and just do two or three exercises per session at the very beginning: try doing only the leg exercises one session, arms and back the next, and chest and shoulders the next. Eventually, beginners will want to do all ten exercises in one session, three sessions a week, because your progress will blossom in direct correlation to the intensity of the challenge. Search online in Google, Yahoo or other search engine for videos demonstrating the exercises by entering the terms set on boldface below.

Perform These 10 Exercises For Beginners' Overall Physique Development:

1. **Dumbbell Shoulder Press**.
2. **Dumbbell Chest Press**, also called **Dumbbell Bench Press**, both arms at once, or one arm at a time.
3. **Push-ups**, from the floor, or a railing.
4. **Ab Crunches**, on the floor.
5. **Chin-ups**, also called Pull-ups, assisted by a stool if necessary.
6. **Chair Squat**, or **Sissy Squat** with no weights, with one hand on back of chair for balance.
7. **Calf Raises** on stairs, unweighted or holding one dumbbell and using the other hand to grab rail for balance.
8. **Leg Lunges**, with or without dumbbells
9. **Dumbbell Biceps Curls**
10. **Dumbbell Triceps Extensions**, one arm at a time.

Again, use a search engine, entering the terms you see above in boldface type into the search field to find videos and instruction. You will find many variations. Chin-ups can be done wide-gripped, close-gripped, palms facing you, or facing away from you. In the beginning, it doesn't matter. Only when you become more advanced will you have the need to fine-tune your workout.

If you find two different videos for the same exercise, but each instructor is doing it differently, try each one and decide for yourself. That's what we all do.

In the beginning especially, all you need to do is perform basic, non-exotic exercises. When you're ready to move on up the food chain, you can graduate to a one bodypart-per-day program.

Chapter 6
My Workout

My workout is never the same twice, but these exercises form the core of my workout routine.

Abs

I do 2 or 3 of the following, 3 times a week:
—Hanging Leg Raises
—Crunches
—Seated Leg Tucks
—Roman Chair Side Bends
—Ab Wheel

Shoulders

—Overhead Shoulder Press on a machine
—Dumbbell Front Raise
—Dumbbell or cable/pulley Lateral Raise
—Dumbbell Rear Flyes, or Rear Delt Machine

I may add upright cable rows and bent over cable rows depending on time and energy level.

Hamstrings & Glutes

—Lying Hamstring Curl machine, or Lying Dumbbell Hamstring Curl
—Standing Hamstring Curl machine
—Butt blaster machine
—Roman Chair hamstring extension

Calves

—Calf raises on various machines at the gym, standing or sitting, including calf raises performed on the leg press machine meant for quads.

Quads

—Leg Press Machine
—Smith Machine Squats
—Leg Extensions

Biceps

—Machine Curls, single arm
—Preacher Curl Machine, two arms
—Dumbbell Preacher Curls, single arm
—Barbell Preacher Curls
—EZ Bar Barbell Curls, standing, or on a preacher bench
—Cable Curls, one arm or both at once.
I choose three from the above list.

Triceps

—One Arm Cable Push Downs
—Triceps Kick-backs, dumbbell or cable
—Overhead Triceps Extensions, seated
—Flat Bench Triceps Extensions, lying on back
—Overhead Triceps Extensions, lying on a decline bench
—Skull Crusher with an EZ Curl Bar

I do the first two, then choose one more from the remaining list.

Forearms

—Crossover Dumbbell Hammer Curls
—Wrist Curls
—Cable One-Arm Reverse Curls
—Preacher Bench Dumbbell Reverse Curls
—Barbell or EZ Curl Bar Reverse Curls

I perform two forearm exercises from the above list, changing the routine each week.

Chest

—Dumbbell Incline Bench Press, or Hammer Strength incline bench press machine
—Dumbbell Flat Bench Press, or Hammer Strength flat bench press machine
—Dumbbell Decline Bench Press, or Hammer Strength decline bench press machine
—Dumbbell Pullover
—Decline Barbell Bench Press
—Cable Standing Flye
—Single Arm Machine Flyes

I always do one each of the first three exercises, then add to the list depending on energy level.

Back

—Cable Lat Pulldowns to the front, or manual pull-ups on chin-up bar
—Bent Over Cable Reverse Flyes
—Seated Cable Rows
—Dumbbell Shrugs, Shrug Machine or Smith machine for trapezius muscle development.
—Single Arm Dumbbell Rows, with one knee on bench
—Smith Machine Deadlifts
—Machine Rows, on whatever machine is available.

I use **Flexsolate** straps for many of my back and shoulder exercises, Flexsolate straps allow your hands to rotate in a natural torque as you perform many exercises, such as Cable Lat Pulldowns to the front. Grasping the bar in the usual way, your hands are fixed firmly in place, producing great stress on the shoulder joints and wrists. The Flexsolate straps disengage the hands from the exercise entirely and allow them to rotate naturally during the execution of the pull-down, thereby stressing the back muscles much more directly.

Flexsolate straps' intended purpose is right in line with all the preaching I have done here about your hands being superfluous to the execution of the exercise. By literally removing your hands from the exercise, these straps allow you to isolate your target muscle in ways not possible using sheer will power alone.

They are excellent for a wide variety of exercises, especially cable rows.

Flexsolate straps come with a demonstration tutorial DVD: <www.flexsolate.com>

For some of my exercises the more traditional style lifting straps are more applicable, and basic styles are cheaply available at Sears, Wal-Mart or most in-gym boutiques for about $7.

A1 Supplements often gives these away for free with a supplement order. A-1 Supplements has the best price on my preferred IsoPure whey protein, and offer cheap shipping to Alaska and Hawaii:
<www.a1supplements.com>

Conventional straps work better for me when doing dumbbell rows or performing shrugs on the trap machine or with dumbbells. I prefer Schiek Model 1000-PLS Power Lifting Straps:
<www.schiek.com/straps.html>

Lifting gloves will save wear and tear on your hands and make the entire workout more comfortable. We're not working out for the purpose of tearing up our hands, or to fatigue them even before our target muscle tires. Keep the stress and focus on the target muscle by cushioning and protecting your hands with workout gloves.

I've bought a lot of gloves, but the best I have found are the Schiek 425 Power Lifting Gloves with Wristwrap. They have embedded gel pods for comfort and wings on the fingers for easy removal after a sweaty workout.
<www.schiek.com/gloves.html>

Chapter 7
The Simple Reclaim Your Youth Diet

"The most effective weight loss exercise is pushing yourself away from the dinner table."
—Advice columnist Ann Landers

Here's the simple, super-special, no-fail Reclaim Your Youth Diet:

You can lose excess weight easily, although perhaps not painlessly, by doing just one of the following:

1. **Eat nothing after dinner**. That means no noshing in front of the TV or computer.

2. **Stop eating between meals**, except for a naked piece of fruit.

3. **Stop eating out**: no fast food places, no diners, no delis, no push-carts, no roach coaches...no restaurants of any kind.

4. **Learn to cook**. The idea that humans have turned over their very survival, and the survival of their own children, to businesses and corporations on whom they have bestowed full responsibility

for feeding them, is *insane*.

An author could theoretically make millions —and many have— by creating and promoting a "brand-new revolutionary" diet, but since the whole idea is mostly hogwash, I doubt I'd be able to fake it well enough to cash in on my share of the market.

When people claim that any given diet has *finally* worked for them, what they are actually saying is that they were finally *psychologically ready* to shed the weight.

Any weight loss diet will "work". All you have to do is stick with it.

The ludicrousness of diet books is their over-complication of a very, very simple problem. You don't need special recipes or elaborate regimens to lose weight. All you have to do is change the way you've been eating, because that's what's made you fat to begin with.

Over-eating is not physical, it's psychological. Being fat has nothing to do with physical hunger, but everything to do with emotional want. Nobody continually stuffs themselves full of food because they have an accelerated nutritional need. They stuff to fill up, and cover up, and build up a protective barrier.

Food is comfort, and no one likes being uncomfortable, so suggesting someone alter their ways means altering their comfort level. And people will naturally balk at that.

I realize I will get nowhere suggesting that people seek professional counseling: and I don't mean from your kindly pastor or a trusted friend. To get to the root of our behavioral problems we need a trained professional who has no emotional ties to us. We need someone who will tell us directly, or make us see, the truth about ourselves. And why we are eating so much crap.

Just as people seem completely mystified that they "gained the weight back" after ending their diet and regressing to the same old eating habits that made them fat in the first place, they are even more puzzled by the idea that unresolved issues in their life are the engine powering their overeating.

After a lifetime of unsuccessfully urging friends and colleagues to get professional counseling —and some of these very people were licensed therapists themselves— I know better than to push such a logical solution. So instead, let's consider something a lot less threatening: making a change in the way we eat.

People like to make very simple scenarios chaotically complicated as a strategy to avoid resolving them. People especially like to pretend they have no idea that they are eating too much food, too often.

Friends from Germany were doing the grand tour of the US one summer by auto, and told me of how they visited a very large and famous BBQ restaurant down south that had dozens of long communal tables completely occupied, and endless herds of big-boned sweaty people lined up outside waiting for an opening, virtually chewing off their own 4XL T-shirts in anticipation of a meal. They were fascinated by the unashamed public display of gluttony, which coming from a foreign perspective of incredulousness, made the picture all the more vivid and funny. They described people wearing big bibs, picking up entire racks of ribs with both fists, and chowing down as grease and BBQ sauce flowed in copious rivers down their hands and arms to their elbows, forming little lakes on the table…and nobody paused to clean themselves off. Sounds kind of gross, but the way they told the story with their German accents, and their sheer disbelief at what they were seeing, made it hilarious.

Advice columnist Ann Landers once said "The most effective weight loss exercise is pushing yourself away from the dinner table."

Chapter 8
What Do I Eat?

The question people ask me most often, after "How old are you?", is "What do you eat?"

It's a fair question because I maintain low bodyfat and people seem to think I have some secret diet or a solution for why I don't appear to have too much trouble maintaining a younger man's physique at my age. I don't call this chapter "My Diet", because for most people, the word diet defines a *temporary* way of eating.

This isn't temporary; it's my everyday way.

The only secret I have is that no food tastes better to me than having a great body feels.

Good health feels great as well, but people will rarely compliment you on your good health. However, they do notice the body.

Additionally, I know which favorite foods of mine are lower in fat grams and calories than others, and I only buy those favorite foods when I shop.

I Only Eat Food That I Like

I don't like rice cakes, but I love rice. I am not crazy about old-fashioned oatmeal, or instant oatmeal, but I love the one-minute variety. I hate cauliflower but like broccoli. Feeling deprived is a sure-fire way to stray from a solid fat-loss or muscle-gain diet. Eating must be enjoyable in order for us to succeed.

I love scallops and I love coconut shrimp, but I only buy the scallops because scallops are far lower in fats and calories than the fried coconut shrimp is. And I never feel deprived when scarfing down caramelized scallops sauteed in a little sesame oil and garlic soy sauce…who would? It's a simple, painless choice.

We all have a choice between foods we like that are low in fat and calories, and foods we like that are high in fat and calories. The mistake many dieters make is they choose to follow a diet that does not allow them to eat foods they like.

You do not need to subscribe to the Atkins diet, or Jenny Craig, or drink canned meal supplements. Devise your own diet using a fat gram and calorie counter book, choosing the foods you like that are lower in calories and fat grams. You'll be able to stick to this kind of custom-designed-for-you diet, based on favorite foods, and adopt it permanently so that you can keep from sliding back into your old eating habits.

The key for me is, I really like the foods I choose, so I'm not eating some repulsive cabbage soup or living on blender meals. I eat foods that I love, but I don't sabotage their health benefits by frying them or by drowning them in butter or creamy sauces.

When I ask my questioners what *they* eat, invariably they speak about foods they just can't give up, or they are "forced" to eat because of lack of time, the kids, etc. They are just making excuses. Their food choices are completely their own, but few people ever own up to that, initially.

One of the best investments you can ever make is a detailed Fat Gram and Calorie Counter book. Buy one that includes restaurant foods if you eat out a lot. Highlight all the foods in the book that you really like but that are also low in fat grams and calories. These foods should make up 97% of your shopping list from now on. Search for these books on amazon.com, then look on the right side of the amazon page for the heading "... Used and New From $00.00". As I write this, good copies of books in this genre can be had for less than a dollar.

We are all individuals, and I have found a personalized nutritional balance between health and fitness that works for me. You need to do the same, through trial and error as I have. If you are overweight, you already know you are eating the wrong foods in portion sizes that are too large.

I know that I cannot snack at night. Ideally, I'd want M&Ms or Wheat Thins if I'm watching TV. But I will absolutely put on fat weight, rather than lean muscle mass weight, if I allow that to become a ritual. I do go through those phases, but I also am quick to recognize that the loss of my goal to look and feel good 24 hours a day is not worth a nightly snack that lasts just a few minutes.

Your personalized plan will entail balancing *calories in* against *calories out* by choosing what to eat and what not, and when. In other words, you will search out the kinds of foods that you enjoy eating in amounts and portions that will not make you gain fat weight.

Metabolism

What exactly is metabolism? Metabolism is our body's action of processing calories, but popularly we use it to refer to fat-burning. Our goal here with *Reclaim Your Youth* is to maintain a level of weight and fitness whereby we achieve an ideal weight and level of fitness, and increase our metabolism, while not feeling deprived in the process.

I am currently exercising at a level that allows me to burn off excess calories, but at the same time I am eating enough of the right kinds of foods to build additional muscle. Simply put, if I increase my calories, but do not increase my exercise activity, I will gain fat weight. If my exercise activity stays the same but I decrease my calories, I will lose both fat and muscle. Overweight people have no consciousness of losing muscle, because they cannot ever see it.

Because I have a good amount of muscle compared to most men my age, I can eat more food without gaining fat weight than they can, because muscle burns fat. The more muscle you have, the more efficiently you burn calories. We can burn a lot more wood, a lot faster, in a big campfire than we can in a small campfire. Think of your metabolism as a campfire; the bigger it is, the more and the faster it will burn calories. I'm not saying you have to become a bodybuilder, because you do not, but if you're fifty years old, male or female, and you have not consistently strength trained during the last 20 years, you have already lost approximately 15% of the original fat-burning muscle mass you once had at age 30.

This is why you may look fatter and softer these days even though you might weigh the same as you did 10 or 20 years ago. Your muscle is disappearing, and along with it your rate of metabolism. You may be getting fatter even though you are not eating more or gaining actual poundage. Your muscle isn't turning into fat; your muscle is disappearing, and being *replaced* by fat.

Resolve to regain your lost muscle, and then some. You will see your life transform completely.

What I Typically Eat, And When

Following is a description of what and when I eat, on average.

Dawn: I drink a glass of water with my statin drug, and I go walk the dogs for 25 minutes.

After the walk, I make a large, very strong frothy skim milk cappuccino with Hershey's powdered cocoa and Splenda, and prepare 2 slices of whole-grain toast with a good amount (3 or 4 tablespoons) of any brand *whole* peanut butter [never Skippy, Jif or other processed kind] and a heaping tablespoon of raspberry preserves. The entire ingredients list for whole peanut butter follows:

—peanuts, salt.

That's it. *Anything* more and it's not real peanut butter.

9 am: 1.5 cups of cooked oatmeal with Splenda and skim milk. I mash a banana into it. I may have other whole grain cereal a couple times a week instead, like Grape Nuts or Raisin Bran.

10 am: 3 or 4 scoops IsoPure protein powder in water with 1 heaping teaspoon Citrucel fiber, 1 level teaspoon creatine monohydrate, and a handful of Dole Mixed frozen fruit, blended into a smoothie. I wash down my supplements with half the smoothie, and pour the other half into a frozen thermos to take to the gym or keep in the fridge if I'm working out at home that day.

Whether I work out at home or go to the gym, I finish the second half of my protein drink after the workout.

2 PM: I grab leftover pasta or stir-fry from the refrigerator from the previous evening's meal and eat it cold out on my lanai with my dogs and the geese.

If there are no leftovers I make a sandwich of home-cooked turkey or chicken salad with mayonnaise on whole grain bread with a glass of skim milk. Or a big bowl of soup, usually lentil, which I make myself from the broth created by stewing a whole chicken. Or I heat up canned low-fat chili with beef or turkey and beans and have that over rice.

6 PM: My favorite dinner is **wild salmon** (as opposed to farm-raised) with the skin on, cooked over medium heat in an undamaged non-stick pan with a little sesame oil. I buy a large slab of salmon and slice it into strips approximately 1.5 inches on each side and 6 inches in length (I freeze what I don't immediately eat), and watch it carefully as it cooks. I set the timer for two minutes, then turn the fish and set the timer again. This gives me a crispy outside and wonderfully rich, fatty, tender interior. I often cook white rice because I love it, although I know brown would be healthier. I sauté a green vegetable like green beans, asparagus or broccoli, with mushrooms and carrots in sesame oil, with chopped garlic and soy sauce on high heat, and may add any other quick-cooking green veggie I have on hand, such as frozen peas, fiddle head fern, or fresh snow peas for the last two minutes of cooking. Everything goes on a plate. Sweet chili sauce from Thailand, salt, and soy sauce go on everything, but sparingly. Just enough for the flavor.

I also like **stir-frys** a lot, slicing chicken breasts or lean beef and sautéing the meat in a non-stick pan, throwing in similar veggies to those above, especially asparagus if I can get it. I make a quick Indonesian peanut sauce with 2 heaping tablespoons natural chunky peanut butter (Adams, Laura Scudder's, or health food store brands), 4 tablespoons sweet chili sauce, 4 tablespoons soy sauce, a good amount of chopped fresh or dehydrated garlic, and 4 tablespoons white wine. I mix this to the consistency of thin chocolate syrup, adding more peanut butter or soy sauce if need be. Then I dissolve I tablespoon cornstarch in a quarter-cup of water or chicken broth and stir the peanut sauce into this.

When the stir-fry is a minute away from being done, I dump in the peanut sauce mixture and stir everything until the sauce coats all the fixin's. Don't walk away. The heat will thicken up the cornstarch fast, and after it has done so, I immediately I pour this dish over rice. If I'm cutting out carbs to cut up a little for an event or photo session, I leave out the rice.

Pasta: I love pasta, all shapes, and I cook it *al dente* and refrigerate what I don't use. I buy quality commercial pasta tomato sauces, whatever's on sale: Paul Newman's, Bertolli, Safeway store brand, Classico. Most are very low in fat and better than I can make myself. I add a little red wine, maybe some mushrooms, always a good amount of garlic. I add cooked chicken breast or 92% fat-free ground beef, browned and drained of excess fat, and sliced zucchini, broccoli or asparagus. Fast and delicious. I always make enough for a couple of additional meals to save time and energy. If I make a lot, I freeze some. When I brown the ground beef in a skillet, I add a cup of water to it when done and cook a few minutes longer, stirring, then drain the water, and the fat along with it, before adding the drained meat to the sauce pot.

I also make **low fat hamburgers** from 92% lean ground beef that I salt beforehand. Again, cook the patty with no oil in an undamaged non-stick pan, but leave it alone: do not smoosh it down with a spatula or anything. If you want a flatburger, form it that way to begin with. Flip after a few minutes. I use Kraft nonfat cheese slices: One slice goes on the bottom of the whole-grain bun, and the other on top of the burger in the pan. It literally takes 20 seconds for non-fat cheese to melt on the burger in the pan, so don't walk away. When the cheese just begins to melt, immediately transfer the burger to the bun. The hot burger will melt the bottom layer of cheese. Top with ketchup and an onion slice or sauteed mushrooms and enjoy. I have made these for many people who loved them and had no idea they were low fat burgers. The secret is; don't squeeze out the juices while the burger cooks. Leave it alone. And don't let the non-fat cheese melt to liquid —this can occur in a matter of seconds. Stand right there and keep an eye on it.

Hot dogs: If I'm being really strict I will eat Ball Park Fat Free brand, which always rate high in taste tests. A delicious alternative with some additional fat is 97% fat-free Hebrew National, which are kosher. I'm not Jewish, but kosher means clean, and I buy kosher *anything* whenever I have a choice. I buy whole grain hot dog buns. I put a single dog on a plate in the microwave on high for 25 seconds. You have to practice with your own microwave to get the timing right. I remove the nuked dog and place it in the bun on top of a nonfat cheese slice. (I tear the cheese slice in half and tuck it down into the crease of the bun.) I wrap the whole thing in a paper towel moistened with a little water to keep the bun soft, and nuke it on high for 30-35 seconds. Make sure the open part of the assemblage faces up so you don't lose all the melted cheese into the paper towel. Unwrap, squirt with mustard and Thai hot chile sauce, and enjoy with ice cold skim milk, or a little wine. A hot dog or two may be an occasional meal.

Another favorite cooking method is to put the hot dog in a little water in my steamer, put the bun in the steamer basket, put the lid on, and cook on high for 2 minutes after it begins to boil. The bun will be very soft and hot. Remove it, open it up and put a slice of fat free cheese in it, plop the hot dog on top, add condiments, and you're good to go.

If I am trying to put on muscle size (which I lose very easily) I eat more muscle-building foods. I like to weigh 180 at 5'9" tall, but can easily fall to 165. To gain the muscle back I need to be very dedicated to eating. It sounds easy, but eating more food than you actually want, and taking the time to make it, takes up a lot of time and mental energy.

I do eat lots of skinless chicken breasts as my main source of protein; the hot dogs and hamburgers are a once a week or less item. I boil a bunch of chicken breasts and use the broth with the fat skimmed off to make lentil soup. I eat the breasts as is, hot or cold, or sliced into spaghetti sauce. Or I saute them in a non-stick pan with a teaspoon of olive oil rubbed on the pan, on low-to-medium flame so the breast is brown on the outside and stays juicy inside. Cook it too fast and it dries out. I eat skinless chicken breasts with steamed broccoli or asparagus more than any other meal. I could add sauces to make it tastier, but I like chicken plain, and sauces add fat, sugar and sodium.

I try not to snack while watching TV, and also rarely eat after 7 PM. I usually have a 6 oz. glass of red wine in the evening. I love it, it's good for the heart, it settles me down, and I sleep like a baby, between the workout drain and the wine-effect. If I need a snack, I open the jar of peanut butter and eat a few spoonfuls with no accompaniment, or spread it on banana or apple slices. I sometimes make cornstarch chocolate pudding using skim milk. My neighbors invite me for a glass of wine weekly, and send me home with goodies once or twice a month that they bake. This is ideal, because if I buy a bag of cookies I will eat them all, but if they give me 3 or 4, that's all I eat, and I'm quite satisfied with that.

I do not eat fast food. I visit McDonald's maybe twice a year, and then it's for grilled chicken breast and a yogurt parfait: no burgers, no fries. I love sushi and that is my favorite fast food. Where I live, in Hilo Hawaii, we have some very high quality yet cheap sushi / sashimi places, so it's an alternative for me that you might not have in your area, or maybe even want. There's also a great bakery near my gym that makes lots of fresh sandwiches on their own whole grain bread, such as real roast turkey, for the same price as fast food. They add a big carrot stick, celery stick and pickle wedge, and one small cookie. For me, it's ideal, fresh, delicious, healthful, filling, with a little sweet snack as a bonus. (Finite portions, like this sandwich box or my neighbors' gift of 4 or 5 cookies, work really well for me.) Subway would be another better alternative to a burger chain.

The above is an example of my seeking out and finding delicious yet low-fat, healthful alternatives to greaseburgers, or fast foods such as Chinese, swimming in fat-laden sauces. Look around in your own area, and ask friends. The usually free-of-cost weekly city alternative newspapers such as the LA Weekly, Honolulu Weekly, San Francisco Bay Guardian, and The Village Voice are some of the best sources for discovering these kinds of inexpensive, healthful eating places.

We all have favorite foods. Some of your favorites, whether you realize it or not, are healthy and contain acceptable levels of fat. Use your fat gram and calorie counter book to search them out. Some of mine are sushi, peanut butter, skinless chicken breasts, mangoes, bananas, roasted almonds, pre-cooked frozen plain shrimp, sauteed scallops. Make your own list, and shop at the market from that. Stay away from the snack aisle.

I don't often eat more food than described here, such as extra snacks, but if I do, I choose food that will take me toward my goal, rather than away from it. For example, brownies don't have the nutrition I need, but Dreyer's 1/2 fat ice cream does. So, if I'm going to eat high-calorie junk, I choose what I call "nutritious junk" that has actual nutritional value...like the ice cream, or a Clif bar instead of oatmeal cookies. Or a Detour Protein Bar instead of a Snickers. They all contain a lot of calories and sugar, but one offers a lot of nutrition I can use, and the other doesn't.

The key is, everything I eat, I really like. I do not ever eat food that I do not enjoy. I do not feel deprived, or as if I'm making some big sacrifice. I am choosing between foods I like that will help me achieve my goal, and foods I like that will not.

If you have a choice between foods you really like that are healthy, low fat/calorie/carb, and will help you accomplish your goal, and other foods you really like that will take you in the opposite direction from your goal, how hard a choice can that be?

You Can't Eat It If It's Not There

I do not often buy tasty snack foods, If I crave chips or chocolate, I buy the smallest bag of Lay's or M&Ms, because I will eat ALL of whatever I buy. An entire Trader Joes Pound Plus Belgian chocolate bar? Gone in less than 24 hours. Santino's corn chips? Gone, the whole bag. Chips Ahoy? Gone, gone, gone. My only solution is to not bring it home from the store.

Realistically, having a body I can be proud of far out-trumps any temporary satisfaction I get from eating tasty snacks. I do binge once or twice a month, but I wouldn't dream of purging. What goes down, stays down.

Muscle And Bone-Building Foods

Incorporating all of these nutrition-charged foods into your diet in place of your present alternatives will fuel your muscle and bone building program:
—Sweet Potatoes
—Fat-free dairy
—Asparagus and broccoli
—Fish
—Chicken and Turkey skinless breast
—Whole grain bread, rice, pasta, etc.
—Eggs
—Oatmeal
—*Moringa*

Dairy (low fat or fat free milk, yogurt, ice cream, cheese, etc.) is essential for bone strength. Eggs are the only animal protein source that is a complete muscle-building protein. Moringa is the only vegetable source that is a complete muscle-building protein.

I have two Moringa trees in my yard. The leaves are protein-packed. The leaves, flowers and seed pods are all highly nutritious. The leaves are delicious but tiny, and very labor-intensive to remove from the fragile stems. I put them in salads and omelets. Moringa can be purchased in Indian/Pakistani markets or easily grown in frost-free climates.

Moringa could save millions from starvation. But until it is better recognized as the miracle food it is, it will not be brought to market in a form we can easily and readily consume. Moringa trees are compact in size, very pretty, require very little water, care, or fertilizer, and my tree grew from seed to 10 feet in less than a year. Entrepreneurs take notice.

So There You Have It

To those who have never restricted their foods before, and never read food labels, my eating routine probably sounds Spartan and regimented. To those who look forward all day long to settling into the sofa come sundown with pizza and beer, and cannot fathom eating a banana instead, I do understand the taste and satisfaction of that particular food choice, but not the frequency, volume, or the short-term and long-term discomfort that results. Not to mention how it impacts your health and looks, and therefore your mood and demeanor.

To wake up suddenly in the night choking on acid reflux and gasping for air is one of the scariest feelings a person can experience. I've been there.

My Mom, in her last 20 years, was preoccupied with food. Every phone conversation or visit centered around talking about food.

While we ate food, she talked about other food she had last week and food she planned to have next week. It was her favorite subject. I feel that there must be an obsessive-compulsive component in this kind of rhapsodic longing for food that seems to increase with age, considering the skyrocketing obesity rates among seniors in America. My mom was still slim and svelte in her mid-50s, but by age 70, she had put on 100 lbs.

I love food, and I genuinely like many of the same foods you do, but I know I can't eat pizza three times a week and not look and feel crappy. Everybody draws the line someplace. If you think it's okay to have pizza three times a week, how did you decide that? Why three times? Why not five? Why not one?

If you drew the line at three, and if you figure out the reasons behind choosing that particular limitation, I think you will discover something very important about yourself, and it will be easier for you to change the way you eat overall without a lot of angst.

I believe that's the key. I love food but I don't dream about it or anticipate it or talk about it so ardently or as eagerly as many people I have known.

I do not feel like I am sacrificing anything by passing by a Baskin Robbins without stopping in. Sometimes I do go in, Most times I don't. I've learned to avoid certain activities with certain friends because they act offended and distanced when I will not scarf down the same amounts of greasy food and drink that they do. I genuinely do not want it. I hate acid reflux, and the idea of taking a drug like Prilosec every day just to accommodate eating greasy junk is insanity to me. My body's telling me I am eating crap because I'm spouting stomach acid. I don't need a ton of bricks to fall on my head.

People never realize how bad they feel until they no longer do.

Chapter 9
**22 Things You Can Do Right Now
To Take Back Your Youth**

> *"We never realized just how well we were doing until we no longer were."*
> —Mary Ellen Sullivan, my grandmother, describing the Great Depression

If you choose just *one* item from the following list, right now, you'll be on your way to applying the brakes to your own individual aging process.

1: Let It Go

Research with centenarians show that the one trait that people who live past one hundred years of age share is the ability to let go and bounce back from adversity. Resilience and the ability to adapt to a changing world seems to have a marked influence on both their staying active and able, as well as their lifespan.

The world is not fair, to be sure, but dwelling on the wrongs of the past interferes with our ability to build a better future. When someone wrongs us, we may be angry about it for a few minutes, or a few years. At some point we're going to stop dwelling on it, so make the decision that you will control what you dwell on, and for how long.

Eventually you're going to let it go anyway, so why not let it go right now?

2: Posture —Play It Straight

Proper posture is a painless way to immediately make an instant and dramatic change in your appearance and demeanor. It can take years off your body's age and add years, or even decades, to the viability of your spine. Most back pain and low back spasms are exacerbated by poor sitting and standing posture.

Good posture will completely transform you. Who among us hasn't been taken aback at some point to realize that reflection they see in a store window of that older person is actually their own?

Stand tall, with your chest out, shoulders back, and stomach in. Stand relaxed, not stiff.

Good posture makes your chest bigger, your tummy smaller and your butt tighter. Holding your head high pulls the facial muscles taut and lessens the volume of a double chin. You grow taller instantly and appear more confident and focused. Your body language says, "Respect me". Your internal organs say "Thank you".

Walking reveals your age by the length of your stride. As we age we take smaller, quicker steps. As you walk, concentrate on stretching each leg further, widening your stride: this is how younger people walk.

3: Banish Trans Fats From Your Diet

Chronic inflammation means your immune system's army is fighting a full-time war. Give it a rest. Reject trans fats, which cause chronic inflammation. Trans fat-free foods taste no different than their evil relations, so this requires no sacrifice on your part. This dietary change requires no deprivation or willpower; you're simply substituting one fat for another.

The words "hydrogenated" or "partially hydrogenated" in the list of ingredients on food labels is your warning not to eat it. The closer the words appear to the beginning of the ingredients list, the more trans fats the food contains. Many foods that claim zero trans fats are not. The government rules allow fudging the truth: if a food claims to be transfat-free, and it has the word "hydrogenated" in the ingredients, it is *not* transfat-free.

Trans fats raise cholesterol and promote heart disease, stroke, cancer and diabetes by inducing chronic inflammation. A dizzying number of convenience and prepared foods contain trans fats. Increasing fiber intake at the same time, such as that found in whole grains and fresh fruits and vegetables, will help trap cholesterol, carcinogens and bacteria and sweep them out of your body before they can get a foothold, lessening the burden on your immune system.

4: Eat Your Breakfast And Pack Your Lunch

Change the stuff you put in your mouth and you will change your body.

People who eat a healthful breakfast have fewer weight control problems than those who skip it. A Harvard study found that people who ate breakfast every day reduced their chances of becoming obese and developing diabetes by 35 to 50 percent compared to people who only ate breakfast twice a week.

Calories ingested at the start of the day are worked off quickly. People who don't eat breakfast will find their blood sugar has plummeted by mid-morning and will be so hungry that they will likely grab the first piece of junk food that comes along, and will go on to make unwise food choices at lunch time.

Don't allow others to decide what goes into your food: pack your lunch instead of buying it. That alone will make your waist narrower and your wallet thicker. Studies have found that restaurant dishes contain an average of more than twice the amount of fat than the same dish prepared at home. Experts at the Kaiser Permanente Center For Health Research found that keeping a food diary, writing down everything you eat and how much, can double your weight loss. Seeing it right there in black and white keeps dieters from "forgetting" how much they've eaten.

The camera may add ten extra pounds to your body, but ten extra pounds on your body adds ten years to your age. Losing excess weight will make you walk and move like a younger person, restore self confidence, make you more attractive and approachable to more people, increase your sexual opportunities and sexual appetite, influence the way you dress, give you more energy, and brighten your mood.

Changing your body will change your life. Just ask anyone who's done it.

5: Drink Enough Water

Eight glasses of water a day? I think it's more important just to maintain hydration evenly throughout the day rather than count glasses of water.

Drink water: lose weight. Our body signals hunger and thirst at the same time, confusing us. Often all it wants is a drink of water, not food. Try drinking a glass of H2O next time you're feeling the urge to snack and see if the hunger signals subside. If you *do* eat, you'll eat less.

Researchers at Stanford University, upon analyzing the diets of 173 overweight women, found that those who drank 6 glasses of water a day consumed about 200 fewer daily calories than those who skimped on water. Often our bodies' signals are misread, and what we think is hunger is often thirst, so next time you feel hungry, especially if it hasn't been that long since you last ate something, have a glass of water first to see if that calms the appetite.

Water helps prevent cavities by moistening dry mouth and washing away food particles embedded between teeth. Water rejuvenates the look and feel of skin, keeps pores freer of blockages that cause zits, brings color to the face, "plumps up" the skin via hydration to keep it looking tighter, fills in small wrinkles, and much more. It even helps us lose weight.

We all know we should drink more water, so why don't we? One reason is because we don't like the inconvenience of having to pee so often. But more visits to the bathroom means that we're getting rid of more of the fats, toxins and other wastes that might otherwise settle into our muscles, skin and internal organs if we don't flush them out. Sure it's inconvenient. But why is it that the same people who eagerly down half a pitcher of Margaritas don't mind four or five tipsy trips to a restroom, and a body that can't function normally, but hate making extra bathroom stops at home when the reward is a body that will function even better than normal? And while we're on the subject, don't fail to flush out the toxins the day after an alcohol binge with enough water to do the job thoroughly.

Instead of seeing the added trips to the bathroom as an inconvenience, see them as a welcome opportunity to shed pounds, take 5 years off your face, save you a trip or two to the dentist, and get rid of the toxins and fats that are making you feel and look old before your time.

6: Stretch

Stretching lubricates connective tissues through the production of chemicals called synovial fluid, inherent in the physical act of stretching itself, resulting in increased suppleness. Stretching relieves tension instantly and allows us to relax both physically and mentally. Stretching in women reduces the severity of dysmenorrhea, or painful menstruation. Stretching in arthritics reduces joint pain. When your muscles are sore from daily tasks or working out, stretching reduces the pain and inflammation…but you must be focused on stretching properly as to not exacerbate the problem.

Perhaps the best outcome of stretching is a renewed sense of body awareness. This is why yoga is so popular and why it has such a long history of proponents. There is a real sense of peace and security that comes from reacquainting yourself with your own body and how it functions, something most of us haven't experienced since we were kids. Being aware of your body will greatly reduce injuries large and small, and make you feel more in control. You will be subjected to fewer aches and pains, and your body will feel years younger.

7: Get Regular And Wash Your Hands

Irregularity adversely affects how big our bellies look. Irregularity can dictate our mood, outlook, stress level, skin clarity, and a host of other things, including that uncomfortable expression on our face. Eating more fresh fruits and vegetables will help a lot, in addition to taking a fiber-based cleanser like Metamucil or Citrucel, or generic psyllium husks, with a full glass of water (which starts the process and keeps it going) every day. Cutting down on fried foods and fatty foods, which act like internal glue, will make a significant difference as well. Drinking water throughout your day will be a great help also.

Scientists estimate that we could have prevented fully three quarters of all the colds and flu we have ever suffered in our lives if we had only washed our hands more often and just kept our fingers out of our mouths. Keep a nail clipper handy. Less flu and colds mean less sick days; less lost wages and business, and less money spent on medicines, doctors and DVD rentals.

8: Beg, Borrow Or Steal An Orthopod

If you're one of the approximately one in two adults over 40 experiencing chronic back pain and see no end in sight, you can reclaim your youth by shaving a couple of decades or more off the way you feel with an Orthopod, or similar apparatus.

If you suffer from virtually any kind of ongoing back pain or ache, this miracle machine will change your life, as it has mine. The Orthopod is also known as the Invertapod. In my early 30s I found I couldn't walk more than 4 or 5 blocks without a severe lower backache setting in due to degenerating discs. Even worse, my sciatica episodes were becoming more cripplingly painful and prolonged. My chiropractor lent me this simple apparatus, and within a couple of days I felt reborn. Years of ache and agony were left behind me.

There is no exercise or exertion whatsoever required with the Orthopod.

With gravity weighing us down and compressing our spine during most of our waking hours, it makes sense that stretching and elongating the spine will relieve the compression, the energy drain, and the stress. This is what this elegantly simple gizmo does. You can reclaim a couple decades of your youth within a few days by using an Orthopod.

Another similar product is called The Total Back System, and can be seen on this website:

http://www.momentum98.com/totalback.html

Orthopods are difficult to come by but may be available as a rental from a hospital supply house. See if it works for you before investing money in a purchase. Many gyms have a similar simple apparatus that allows you to stretch your spine with the body's weight *supported at the hips*.

Hanging upside down from the ankles is not only scary, but also physically impossible for most people. The fear most people have is, because they are weak and sore to begin with, they will not be able to return to an upright position and will become trapped.

Inversion tables impede a full stretch; hanging freely from the hips gives a far superior elongation and allows the subject to flex and bend the spine to work out kinks, while feeling safe. So an Invertapod, or similar machine, that pivots and supports your weight at the hips, is the ideal anti-gravity machine.

You do not even need to pivot completely upside down to achieve a beneficial result from the Orthopod or similar. I often keep my feet firmly planted on the floor as I bend over the supporting cushion, for the simple relief that position alone offers.

9: Read

Information evolves continually, daily, even minute-by-minute. Reading has rewarded all of us with valuable knowledge and by revealing new opportunity countless times in our pasts, and will continue to do so in the future. Internet search engines are the greatest boon to human knowledge in history. Website message boards, forums and blogs can allow people with common interests or problems to share their feelings and find solutions. Read newspapers, books, free local periodicals, and food packaging. Reading is knowledge, and knowledge is power. Knowledge is everywhere, and most of it is free for the taking.

10: Fix Yourself

Millions of people walk around in a state of unrehabilitated "minor" injury on a daily basis, and do little to fix themselves. Others are much too casual about taking prescribed medications for serious treatable or preventable maladies. Whenever we suffer an injury and choose pain-masking pills, denial or "toughing it out" over recuperation, rehabilitation or surgery, we are choosing to get old before our time.

Poor vision, garbled hearing, decaying teeth, problem knees, backs, shoulders, elbows and the like all mean we can do less, less often, and with less vigor. Allowing blood pressure, pre-diabetes condition or other treatable problems to get out of control via denial or apathy is quite simply, insane, considering the gravity of the problems that are certain to ensue.

Those with ongoing physical injuries need to see a doctor who has a specialty in that particular body part. Physical Therapists are the true strength training professionals, and the fact that so many injured people do not see a Physical Therapist who can get them back to full mobility is hard to understand. Perhaps not every problem can be fixed 100%, but a marked improvement in most individuals' quality of life is more the rule than the exception. Many injuries can be cleared up can just by following doctors' recommendations and a sound rehabilitation program with a Physical Therapist. Once the PT teaches you what to do, many physical rehab programs can be carried out all by yourself at home.

When I am in Los Angeles and I see people jogging in bumper-to-bumper traffic, deeply breathing in carbon emissions, and the same people are also wearing a brace on their knee because of an injury, I don't see health or fitness, I see blind stupidity.

If it hurts, stop. Rest, recuperate, recover.

11: Change Doctors

A good doctor is worth his weight in hundred dollar bills. A bad doctor can make you old before your time, and then kill you.

Hardly a soul reading this does not know about a friend or relative who was misdiagnosed, ignored, or medically mistreated by his or her doctor. If your doctor rushes you out before you have a full understanding of things, is condescending, tells you it's "all in your head", can't keep his balance because his own head is too big, or simply doesn't listen to you, then it's time to make a change.

Older patients continually encounter ageism. A doctor will tell someone in their 60s or 70s that their pain or diminished capacity is simply due to age, and should just be accepted. However, a patient in his 20s presenting with identical symptoms, to the same physician, will be aggressively treated.

Good doctors are out there. Keep searching. Don't solely rely on one doctor to recommend another. Even if your primary care physician is sending you to a specialist for your problem, ask around and do some research on that choice. The best recommendation for a good doctor comes from a satisfied, much improved patient, not a crony.

12: Stop Smoking And Benefit Instantly

Within minutes of quitting, a smoker's risk of sudden death from heart attack begins to diminish, so forget that excuse about "it's too late for me…the damage has already been done".

Within hours of stopping, the chronic inflammation caused by incessantly burning your throat and lungs can begin to heal, lessening the risk of major disease and heart attack.

Within a day of stopping, your body begins to cleanse itself of toxins; carbon monoxide is banished, nicotine disappears from the blood and oxygen flow is increased. Within weeks of quitting, you cough less, you can taste and smell once again, and cilia regrow, sweeping mucous, toxins and solid pollution particles from your bronchial tubes and throat.

The single best thing you can do for your health and longevity is to quit smoking. Smoking makes you look and feel old and sick long before your time. It ravages skin color and texture and creates deep wrinkling. And your smoke screen repels the very people who can help you stay young: those you love. It took a while for you to learn how to smoke, so cut yourself some slack when attempting to quit. Just keep trying.

13: Include Dietary Supplements

Perhaps one person in a hundred gets all their daily necessary nutrients from the food they eat, so despite the constantly flip-flopping of professional opinions pertaining to the efficacy of multi-vitamins, a good multi-vitamin is a benefit for all of us.

Yes, we know about studies that claim a multi-vitamin is only just as effective as a placebo. But these studies continually contradict each other and cause untold confusion, making many of us just throw up our hands in resignation. Taking a multivitamin is just common sense, especially if your diet is lacking in fruits and vegetables. The amount of folic acid in the average commercial multi vitamin, for example, has been shown to slash colon cancer odds by 60% in men. A Harvard University study showed that women who took multivitamins containing folic acid over a 15-year period cut their colon cancer risk by 75%.

Growing muscle requires increased protein. Drinking a high quality protein shake within forty-five minutes of your chosen workout will maximize your workout benefits, speed your recovery, and more quickly create the results you're working toward. We can increase calcium intake via dairy product consumption, and a good supplement will add to the bone-building benefits that strength training brings. Anti-oxidants may help protect against cancer, and Omega-3 and Omega-6 fatty acids, which are found in salmon, nuts, fish oil and flaxseed oil for example, help your heart and your brain.

But remember, when it comes to supplements, more is not better. Stick to the recommended dosages.

14: Hormone Replacement Therapy

Hormone Replacement Therapy is simply the replenishment of the hormones your body used to produce naturally as a matter of course, but no longer does. Whether male or female, HRT can significantly improve mood and outlook, sexual drive and function, skin and muscle condition, and a host of other things. Most people report that HRT makes them feel younger and more alive again. HRT can go a long way in relieving depression, banishing aches and pains, and increase energy and stamina.

Female HRT has increasingly fallen from favor due to connections with increased forms of cancer and heart disease; it isn't for everyone due to individual medical constraints, so consult a hormone specialist to see if HRT may be right for you in your case.

Testosterone replacement in men can go a long way in helping reclaim youthfulness. Testosterone therapy can alleviate or banish depression, imbue a feeling of overall well-being, restart libido, add lean muscle mass, speed healing from physical injury large or small, improve skin tone and texture, to list a few benefits.

Male HRT, such as testosterone replacement, is not recommended for those with a history of cancer. For those with a family history of heart disease, testosterone replacement may cause an increase in red blood cell production, making it more difficult for your heart to pump the thickened blood. Donating blood once a month may be the answer to this particular dilemma for some.

The majority of men and women over age 50 have lost their full ability to produce essential hormones. Some family doctors and general practitioners can be HRT-resistant for various reasons other than medical, including prejudice, or just simple ignorance of the science.

HRT Specialists will have a fuller knowledge and understanding of each individual's unique requirements. HRT can have its risks, some of them not fully substantiated, so consulting a specialist and doing your research to ascertain what is right for you are essential.

15: Shoot Yourself

Or ask a friend to do it for you, and forget that the video camera's there. Set it up on a tripod to shoot yourself doing housework, interacting with family or friends, working at the office or playing with the dog. See yourself move, stand and speak as others see you, off-guard. It will be a revelation. Those tapes of you all dressed up at that birthday or wedding with your stomach temporarily pulled in and wearing your best camera face...they don't count.

Viewing ourselves as others see us can be unsettling. But there's nothing like seeing ourselves in an unflattering light, and realizing that others see us that way all the time, to shock us into making rapid changes for the better.

16: Take Control of Something You Actually *Can* Control

Right at this moment, all of us are enjoying the exact kind of body and overall general health that we have worked toward all our lives, for better or for worse.

Every decision pertaining to what we have consumed and inhaled and what our level of activity has been over our lifetime has resulted in the very body we inhabit and the level of health we enjoy at this moment. Our bodies will continue to change and evolve in positive or negative ways according to the future decisions we make.

Denying that we have a problem delays a solution, accelerates our downhill slide, and exacerbates the predicament. In order to begin to change our lives in a positive way we have to take responsibility for our decisions: denying what we eat, how much, and how often doesn't mask the problem. People who make jokes about their junk food intake and low level of physical activity are doing themselves a great social disservice by making public light of the low regard in which they hold themselves.

It is always enlightening to see interviews on TV with people before and after an extraordinary weight loss. The level of denial, defensiveness and the rejection of personal responsibility expressed in the "before" interview is dramatically different from the generally balanced assessment and acceptance of responsibility revealed once the problem has been resolved.

17: Breathe Deep, And Exhale Even Deeper

Many of us spend all our waking hours literally waiting to exhale. If we pay close attention, chances are we'll often catch ourselves holding our breath throughout our day, especially during stressful episodes.

Just as muscle atrophies with age, so does lung capacity. Beginning in our mid-20s, non-smokers lose 10% of their lung capacity every decade. That's really unsettling. A non-smoker in his or her mid-seventies may have lost fully half their lung capacity. Smokers lose even more. If we are not consciously working at increasing our breathing capacity, then we are losing breathing capacity.

Just as regulating the amount of water we drink will flush toxins and impurities from our bodies, so will proper breathing techniques. The problem is not just that we don't inhale deeply enough, it's that we don't exhale fully either. Our rib cages have expanded, and become fixed that way, because we never expel enough air from our lungs to allow the rib cage to contract as fully as it's supposed to. In older people, this can contribute to the "barrel-chest" look. Consciously pushing air out of our lungs, expelling as much trapped stale air as we can, will make room for new, fresh, cleansing, oxygen-rich, microbe-killing air.

Many of us breathe via our stomachs and not our chest. Look down as you breathe normally…what expands as you inhale, your upper chest or your tummy? If it's your tummy, you're breathing wrong. And most of us are guilty of doing it.

Breathing purposely, regularly and fully will instantly relax our entire being. Proper, purposeful breathing increases oxygen in the blood and lowers blood pressure. When our blood is heavily oxygenated it becomes more difficult for bacteria and viruses to grow in our bodies; injuries and wounds heal faster, we recover from sickness more quickly and muscle growth is enhanced.

18: Seek Calm

The media loves to tell us how busy we all are these days, how hectic our lives have become. The media also fills the airwaves with fear and loathing-inducing stories that have an enormous dehumanizing and desensitizing effect upon us, our friends and our loved ones.

"Commentators" with their own shows or prominent spots on others', regale with their lies, rumors and half-truths, addressing a huge audience *hungry for chaos and turmoil*. What does that say about people, when after a long stressful day they settle into their easy chair to faithfully watch some bloated and angry old Irish guy froth at the mouth over matters real or imagined?

When I moved from Los Angeles to rural Hawaii in 2004, I made a conscious decision: no more cable or broadcast TV.

I had known for some time the negative, demoralizing and dunning effect it had on me to keep the TV on in the background, subconsciously absorbing all the negativity that drives the American media.

I now receive no signal on my TV: I watch DVDs. My news comes from internet sites where I can choose what I watch or read, rather than having it fed to me intravenously.

Reject chaos and the unbalanced beings that feast upon it. To choose an activity that ties one's stomach in knots over taking a nap, or building something in the basement, or going to the gym, as millions do, is quite literally, crazy.

Our daily routine is ultimately under our own control despite the obligations we've given permission to entangle us, whether we're ready to admit that or not. We often fill our lives with frenetic activity for the same reasons we fill our stomachs continuously with comfort food…to assuage emotional emptiness and to keep from having to deal with the real problems in our lives. We feel compelled to take on unnecessary activity or the perceived problems of others just so we can evade our own issues, and only *we* can apply the brakes. Learn to say no.

The best way to seek calm is obvious: sleep. If you have trouble sleeping, try supplementing with tryptophan, or try warm milk, or save your glass of wine for bedtime. Shut off your mind. Steal a nap whenever you can.

Some people might dismiss even the easiest suggestions on this list because they're "too busy". But we have all experienced getting caught up in doing time-consuming things that are both unnecessary and which provide little added value to our lives, while rejecting the simple and nearly effortless things, like many of those included in this chapter, which can improve our daily lives.

19: Have A Glass Of Wine With Dinner

If you do not have a history of alcohol problems, partaking in a glass of red wine with dinner or in the evening is not only rife with health benefits, but is a great way to unwind from the day's stresses. Wine opens up arteries and increases blood flow, which has a positive effect in the case of heart disease. It has been determined that a glass of red wine a day can lower your risk of dying from heart disease by 30% to 40%. Moderate wine drinkers are less likely to develop macular degeneration, the age-related eye condition that can lead to partial blindness. Moderate wine drinking increases the levels of HDL, the "good" cholesterol. Red wine prevents LDL, the bad cholesterol, from damaging artery walls. Moderation is very important since alcohol infuses every cell, and its overuse damages our genes and inflames our livers.

20: Get Stronger

If we're not consciously working at getting stronger, then we're actually becoming weaker with every passing day.

Getting stronger means building muscle. Our lean muscle mass acts as a 24-hour a day fat-burning furnace, and is not only the key to more effortless fat-loss and weight control, but is the very place where our immune system resides. The greater our lean muscle mass, the stronger and more efficient will be our ability to fight germs, bacteria, viruses, and disease.

For long term, life-long success at weight control, especially for people with a history of obesity or yo-yo dieting, strength training provides the soundest base from which to rebuild their metabolic foundation. The more lean muscle mass one has, the greater the rate of metabolism. The greater your metabolism, the more efficiently your body burns fat, with less effort.

It's far more crucial for older people to strength train than it is for younger people, simply because older people have already lost a significant amount of precious lean muscle mass —about 7%

for each decade past age 30. Sufficient muscle mass makes our legs strong and keeps us from falling down. Muscle mass is the foundation of an efficient immune system. Muscle mass is what makes a beautiful body, male or female, *beautiful*. Muscle mass burns excess fat. Muscle mass allows for explosive movements, which can save our lives and those of our loved ones in emergencies.

Seniors don't just start losing their balance and breaking hips because they're old. They fall because their muscles have weakened to such an extent that they can't lift their feet high enough to clear even the lowest obstacle. They fall because their muscles are so depleted that their legs turn to noodles and they collapse while just standing there. The hips break on impact because they've lost a crucial amount of bone density. Whoever said that people should slow down and take it easy once we get older had it completely backwards. The older we get, the more essential it is that we strength train.

After middle age, women can benefit from strength training even more than men. Bone loss affects far more women than men. Strength training doesn't just stop bone loss, it actually grows brand-new bone. Strength training also improves balance, minimizing the possibility of falls. Science has proven we are never too old to build new muscle and bone, even well into our nineties.

As an added perk, strength training can give you the beautiful body you've always wanted by building, shaping and sculpting your arms, legs, back and other body parts into a work of art of your choosing and under your control.

You need not be obsessive about working out to get impressive results; you just have to be consistent.

Although not as transforming as strength training, you can begin getting stronger in small, simple ways right now, by taking the stairs instead of the elevator (the engine for stair climbing should be in your buttocks, not your knees), walking more quickly and taking longer strides than normal, or taking the long way around instead of a shortcut. Canadian researchers found that people who participate in regular moderate exercise increase their body's production of immunoglobulin A, the immune system enzyme that fights the common cold. The Centers for Disease Control and Prevention state that people who spend 10 minutes a day walking up and down stairs can lose as much as 10 pounds over the course of a year with no change in their diet.

Now, if you're ready for a real long-term commitment, consider rescuing a dog. I didn't really get to know my own neighborhood —or my neighbors— until I started walking my new dog. Rain or shine, too cold or too hot, I have to walk him and his new brother whether I feel like it or not. And as much as I like to whine about it, the benefits to all of us have been undeniable. If you have a lifestyle that allows sufficient time and love for a dog, both your lives will benefit enormously.

21: Never Retire

Even if you hate your job and know exactly how much time you have left to the day, view that ending as a new beginning. Many policemen and firemen, for example, can retire with a pension after 20 years, while still in their early forties, allowing a new chapter to open in their still-youthful lives. But no matter how old you'll be when your present career ends, consider starting a new one soon after, whether it pays you a salary or not. The most rewarding and successful businesses are always those that incorporate the best-loved interests of the owner.

Fresh goals are what keep us going. Always have more than one future goal, more than one event or milestone that you can get excited about and anticipate. Boredom and lack of purpose lead to depression, and this ugly combination may have you asking why you're still bothering to hang around. We all need purpose, and the beauty of "retirement" is that we are then free to take up any endeavor we wish, whether it's joining the Peace Corps, teaching on a formal or casual level, volunteering, or making good money doing something we'd gladly do for free anyway. Or if you love what you're doing for a living already, why stop?

Those who are still computer illiterate have diminished their world in the most extraordinary kind of way. The first sign that you're getting old is one's turning away from new technology. You can do business on the Internet without anyone seeing how old you are, how you dress, or what you look like. Making money in your underwear is a very empowering thing.

22: Lie About Your Age

The most diabolical force launching us headlong toward old age is our own permission.

Buying into Old Age includes worrying about it, obsessing over it, getting depressed about it, regretting things we did or failed to do, becoming fearful, and the final nail in the coffin —so to speak— giving up on youthful endeavors and abandoning fresh goals.

We have a choice whether or not to embrace all the old wives' tales, our older friends' and relatives' personal horror stories, and the societal stigmas that are projected upon us. A Yale University study showed that those with a positive view of growing older lived on average 7 years longer than those who complained or obsessed about it.

So cut yourself some slack. The next time you forget something, understand that it's nothing new, not necessarily a "senior moment", nor a sign of early Alzheimer's. We've all been forgetting stuff regularly since we were little kids.

My mom taught me something when she turned 80: she said that although we may feel a little frayed on the outside, in our minds we're always still 12, or 18, or 35. We still *feel* those ages because we *own* those ages. We have had a full year's experience being each of those ages, and every age in between, and those ages will always be a part of the fabric of us.

We're never too old to begin something brand new. We're never too old to begin a new relationship or get the hell out of a toxic one, to move to a new city, country, or better climate, or make other life changes that will initiate a major difference in our outlook and happiness.

That 20 year old who still lives inside us would approve.

-end-